W0232692

Houses of Madness

Houses of Madness

Insanity and Asylums of Bengal
in Nineteenth-century India

DEBJANI DAS

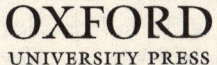

OXFORD
UNIVERSITY PRESS

OXFORD
UNIVERSITY PRESS

Oxford University Press is a department of the University of Oxford.
It furthers the University's objective of excellence in research, scholarship,
and education by publishing worldwide. Oxford is a registered trademark of
Oxford University Press in the UK and in certain other countries

Published in India
by Oxford University Press
YMCA Library Building, 1 Jai Singh Road, New Delhi 110 001, India

© Oxford University Press 2015

The moral rights of the author have been asserted

First Edition published in 2015

All rights reserved. No part of this publication may be reproduced, stored in
a retrieval system, or transmitted, in any form or by any means, without the
prior permission in writing of Oxford University Press, or as expressly permitted
by law, by licence, or under terms agreed with the appropriate reprographics
rights organization. Enquiries concerning reproduction outside the scope of the
above should be sent to the Rights Department, Oxford University Press, at the
address above

You must not circulate this work in any other form
and you must impose this same condition on any acquirer

ISBN-13: 978-0-19-945887-5
ISBN-10: 0-19-945887-1

Typeset in Adobe Garamond Pro 10.5/13
by Tranistics Data Technologies, New Delhi 110 019
Printed in India by Rakmo Press, New Delhi 110 020

To
Kublai and Kopsia

CONTENTS

ILLUSTRATIONS

FIGURES

MAPS

TABLES

ACKNOWLEDGEMENTS

THE COMPLETION OF THIS BOOK would have been impossible without the constant assistance, guidance, and support of many who have patiently been by my side all these years. I would like to take this opportunity to dearly and sincerely thank them all. I am especially grateful to my supervisor, Professor Tanika Sarkar, for her incisive comments and invaluable suggestions. Her insistence that I discuss, analyse, write, and rewrite at every stage helped me to explore a wide range of possibilities. I am thankful to Dr Biswamoy Pati, Dr Mridula Ramanna, Professor Kunal Chakrabarti, and Professor Deepak Kumar for their valuable suggestions and comments.

Adopting the assistance of different disciplines is an essential tool and I wish to thank my friend Kausik Ghosh at the Department of Geography and Environment Management, Vidyasagar University, for drawing the maps in this book. I would also like to thank my colleague Kaushik Ghosh, architect and urban planner, for drawing the diagrams, which will help readers have an idea of the nineteenth-century asylum plans. A word of sincere thanks also to the publisher, copy-editor, and two reviewers whose suggestions helped me a lot.

I am grateful to the staff and archivists of the West Bengal State Archives, Kolkata; the National Library, Kolkata; Bangiya Sahitya Parishad, Kolkata; the National Archives of India, New Delhi; the Teen Murti Library, New Delhi; the Central Secretariat Library, New Delhi; the National Medical Library, New Delhi; Jawaharlal Nehru University,

New Delhi; the British Library, London; and the Wellcome Library, London.

I am indebted to my parents, my parents-in-law, and to my sister-in-law, Manjusha. I would like to take this opportunity to dearly thank my friends, including Mamta, Uma, Sarani, Jagori, Shewli, Sovanjan, and Subhajit, who were there patiently by my side through all the ups and downs and have accepted me the way I am. I am also lovingly thankful to Timur, who silently cheers me up at all times. Discussions with my friends Shilpi Rajpal and Erica Wald have always been encouraging; their comments and suggestions have made me rethink my work on several occasions. I also take this opportunity to thank my colleague Gautam Chando Roy in whom I have found a wonderful friend. Through several discussions, he has made me think about aspects of social history, which have helped me immensely. He constantly supports, encourages, and inspires me to think, write, and do research.

Any work can never excel without positive and discerning criticisms. Deep Kanta, my husband, is my best critic. Discussions with him have always been the most knowledgeable experience. He always makes me think and question my work, and I have benefitted greatly from him.

My final and greatest debt is to my brother, Dhiman, without whom neither would I have thought of writing this book nor would I have been what I am today.

INTRODUCTION

Yes!
Mental Illness is Treatable
Mental Health Week
(Advertisement, *Times of India*, 8–14 December 2010, New Delhi edition)

THIS ADVERTISEMENT IN A NEWSPAPER was published by the Government of India along with a week-long schedule of mental illness awareness campaigns. Its various activities included painting competitions, poster exhibitions, and street plays highlighting issues surrounding mental illness and discussions on 'identification and management of common mental diseases'. This showed the government's initiative to address mental illness and also to make its citizens aware of the malady, which is curable. Also, by publicizing the event, the government made an effort to break the taboo associated with mental illnesses in India. It reached out to the maximum number of people through several programmes based on community engagements. It assured the public that mental illness was curable like any other disease. Such an awareness campaign, there-fore, highlighted the beneficial measures adopted by the government to address issues of mental health. It also showed the need to control and curb problems related to it. In the present day, mental illness is a cause of alarm as many people, both in developed and developing countries, are increasingly being diagnosed with the problem. In post-Independence India, issues of mental health were addressed not only in mental hospitals or psychiatric institutions, but also through several non-governmental organizations; for instance, in recent years, two very significant non-governmental organizations working on community mental health problems are The Banyan Tree in Chennai and Iswar Sankalpa in Kolkata. In the treatment of mental illness, the difference between the functioning of a government-run institution and a non-governmental organization is that while the former particularly limits itself to the treatment of patients once they are admitted, the latter engages itself more with the community at large. In doing so, these organizations try to reach out to the community, take initiatives to locate homeless persons suffering from mental illnesses, admit them at their treatment shelters, and at the end of the treatment regime, not only take steps to return the patients to their families but also very effectively continue with their post-treatment care. Mental patients are admitted into such homes or shelters either by their family members or by the police. The government's engagement with the issue and the gradual involvement of non-governmental organizations emphasize the relevance and need for awareness of mental illness even in the present day.

While the Indian government of the twenty-first century attempted to bring mental illness to public attention by putting an advertisement in a local newspaper, the authorities in the nineteenth century kept it a private affair within the closed walls of asylums. Though the present-day government makes an effort not to associate mental illness with any taboo or shame, but to recognize it as a disease that is curable if treated on time, the colonial government tried to cover up the subject as it not only conceived mental illness as a matter of pity and hopelessness but also did not recognize it as a curable disease until the end of the nineteenth century.

'Insane hospitals' or 'lunatic asylums' were terms used in medical records of the nineteenth century to define institutions where mentally ill individuals were confined. Patients were admitted into those institutions either by their family members, friends, acquaintances, or by the police, but always under the supervision of the Magistrate of the state. A look into the period reveals various attempts by medical officers of both the East India Company and the colonial government to understand mental illness. The nineteenth century witnessed the evolution of several definitions of insanity and the insane, including experiments on asylum construction. This also led to the proliferation of asylums in India.

In particular, this book studies the reasons for the environmental and geographical locations of the asylums of Bengal. It further analyses how that determined the architecture of asylums and the method of treatment within them. During the nineteenth century, the definition of insanity was constantly revised and reframed. Within this context, gender issues played a key role: it became difficult for the medical practitioners to situate 'mad' women. Even though medical officials found it problematic to define them, possibly because of the relatively small number of women admitted into asylums, they still constructed an image of insane women that needs to be questioned.

In Europe and America, a whole body of scholarly work exists and is still being produced on insanity and mental asylums. These address a range of issues from treatises on insanity and its definitions to the condition of patients in the asylums and the acts and policies implemented. Medical literature written by physicians in England and America during the early nineteenth century is also extensive. In India, the issue of insanity in the nineteenth century has not been extensively dealt with, other than very important contributions made to the field by Waltraud Ernst and James Mills.[1] The present work is a new contribution to the already expanding historiography of colonial psychiatry, as it takes up the case of the Bengal Presidency, which was very important with Calcutta being the capital of British India during the nineteenth century. It was here that the first European Lunatic Asylum was established along with several other 'native' asylums, much before they were constructed in any other part of India. Although there is an extensive literature on the issue in general, there is a particular dearth of historiography on the area in the case of Bengal; hence, much of this work is based on primary sources and their interpretations. Since English and European physicians were in charge of the asylums in Bengal, the medical literature and references drawn in this work are also based on their observations on what was happening in England and how they tried to translate their knowledge into practice in Bengal.

This work concentrates on the nineteenth century as it was the period when various definitions of insanity evolved, asylums were built in India,

---

[1] Waltraud Ernst, *Mad Tales from the Raj: European Insane in British India, 1800–1858* (London: Routledge, 1991); James Mills, *Madness, Cannabis and Colonialism: The 'Native Only' Lunatic Asylums of British India, 1857–1900* (Basingstoke: Macmillan, 2000).

rules and regulations were made, and acts on lunacy were also passed to govern the mentally ill. In England, the beginning of parliamentary enquiries on madhouses began in 1807, followed by an act to set up public asylums in 1808. Porter has pointed out that there has been 'no attempt to create an interpretative synthesis of English madness before institutionalization became the dynamo of change in the nineteenth century'.[2] Another reason why this study is confined to the nineteenth century is because it marked the consolidation of British rule in India. Therefore, it is also necessary to know whether the transfer of power from the Company to the Crown caused any shift in the understanding of insanity and its treatment as well as in the laws implemented to control those who were mentally unfit.

Michel Foucault's work *Madness and Civilization* is a significant contribution to the field. He argued that Western European culture actually lost some of its reasons or homogeneity by silencing the voices of madness in its midst. Foucault drew his examples from the 'classical age', written about by observers such as Thomas Willis, Robert Whytt, Philippe Pinel, and Samuel Tuke. He explained how asylums and prisons became sites of disciplining and punishing of the self and for 'surveillance and judgement'. Discussing the methods of treatment practised in the asylum, he pointed out that the underlying principle was that 'madness will be punished in the asylum'. The primary concern of the mental hospital was to sever and to 'correct'; therefore, according to him, therapeutics did not function in the infirmary. Methods of treatment such as 'consolidation', 'purification', 'ablution', and 'regulation of movement' were efforts towards disciplining the inmate. Another significant aspect of treatment in the asylum was labour, which, according to Foucault, was enforced to regulate patients into a disciplined workforce. Work in an asylum, according to him,

> is deprived of any productive values; it is imposed only as a moral value; a limitation of liberty, a submission to order, an engagement of responsibility, with the single aim of disalienating the mind lost in the excess of a liberty which physical constraint limits only in appearance.[3]

[2] Roy Porter, *Madmen: A Social History of Mad Houses, Mad Doctors and Lunatics* (Stroud, Gloucestershire: Tempus, 2004), 15.

[3] Michel Foucault, *Madness and Civilization: A History of Insanity in the Age of Reason*, tr. Richard Howard (New York: Vintage Books, 1965), 248.

This work differs from Foucault's views on insanity by arguing that asylums were not only places to 'discipline and punish', but also to understand insanity as a disease and implement various treatments for its remedy. The treatments practised in the asylums were undoubtedly harsh, although the physicians of the time were not skilled enough to put through the precise practice, or to understand what insanity was. This study also shows how labour in the asylums of Bengal had a profit value added to it. Labour in the asylum was considered as both a part of moral treatment and a source of profit for the maintenance of its inmates.

The history of 'colonial psychiatry' has opened up a broad spectrum of subject areas of study in mental illness and asylum practices. Richard Keller has pointed out that the 'European doctors monopolized the medical profession, allowing Indians to initially occupy only the most menial positions in the asylums'.[4] He further stated how 'asylum physicians in Britain advocated work as a means of "moral management" of mental illness'. However, British physicians in India 'found hard labour impracticable, if not injurious to Europeans because of the harsh tropical climate'.[5] This was why Europeans at the European Lunatic Asylum of Bengal were not allowed to do any physical labour, while on the contrary labour was crucial at the 'native' asylums. Thus, issues of race and class were significant aspects in the understanding of insanity in the nineteenth century.

Ernst's work on the European asylums of India focused on issues of race and class divisions in the asylum, providing a different dimension to the understanding of insanity. According to her, asylums were places of 'refuge' or 'temporary receptacles', and 'madness unlike destitution crossed barriers of social class'.[6] The definitions and discourse of mental illness in nineteenth-century British India could not be isolated from the 'social context' in which they existed. She further states that the medical practitioners and the 'administrators utilized social discriminations based on race and class to uphold white supremacy'.[7] Hence, first-class

---

[4] Richard Keller, 'Madness and Colonization: Psychiatry in the British and French Empires, 1800–1962,' *Journal of Social History* 35, no. 2 (Winter 2001): 295–326.

[5] Keller, 'Madness and Colonization,' 295–326.

[6] Ernst, *Mad Tales from the Raj*.

[7] Ernst, *Mad Tales from the Raj*, 115–20.

patients were diagnosed as suffering from 'temporary weakness' while patients of other classes were termed as 'idiots' and 'maniacs'. As most patients belonged to the latter group, asylums operated as last resorts for those European soldiers and poor Whites who did not respond to societal discrimination or military discipline. Europeans were sent back home for further treatment after their temporary stay in asylums in India. This 'repatriation of deranged colonial servants to Britain', according to her, 'brings back home the fact that colonial rule also took its toll on the British'.[8] It also illustrated the Company's 'swift measures to make "invisible" those who might otherwise tarnish the image and self perception of the British as a mentally and physically superior person'.[9]

Gender is an important issue that cannot be ignored in understanding the dynamics within the asylums. Louise Hide's recent work, *Gender and Class in English Asylums, 1890–1914*,[10] deals with the issue of gender and class as it shows how there was a sudden increase in asylum admissions during the Victorian period in England as the result of socio-economic changes that affected people's lives in England during the time. The book also addresses another very important aspect of studying insanity, showing how towards the end of the nineteenth century, certain nomenclatures and the functioning of the asylum changed, as Victorian psychiatry took a 'clinical turn' away from asylums to mental hospitals, and from attendants to nurses. Hide's work further addresses the relationships between doctors, patients, and attendants inside England's asylums through the notions of masculinity and femininity as understood during the time.

Appignanesi in her work *Mad, Bad and Sad* has also provided further insight into the issue of gender, as she has shown how a 'particular period's definitions of femininity or masculinity were closely linked to definitions of madness.'[11] She has demonstrated how diagnoses and

[8] Waltraud Ernst, 'Asylum Provision and the East Indian Company in the Nineteenth Century', *Medical History*, 42, no. 4 (1998): 476–502.

[9] Ernst, *Mad Tales from the Raj*, 166.

[10] Louise Hide, *Gender and Class in English Asylums, 1890–1914* (Basingstoke: Palgrave Macmillan, 2014).

[11] Lisa Appignanesi, *Mad, Bad and Sad: A History of Women and the Mind Doctors from 1800 to the Present* (London: Virago Press, 2008), 7.

explanations of mental illnesses are shaped by different transitions in history; hence, the understanding of mental illness varies from one period to the other. Similarly, Indrani Sen's work on the mental illnesses of the 'white woman' in the colonies established the link between the 'conditions of gendered life in the colony and the problem of mental disorder'. Instead of dealing with the question of 'insanity alone', she concluded that the 'mental disorders' of European women in India was a result of social, economic, and cultural conditions. Sen studied the mental disorders of European women within the context of the distinctions made by present health experts among 'severe' and 'common' mental illness.[12]

Phyllis Chesler in her work *Women and Madness*[13] focuses on the construction of madness within Western patriarchal societies. There was a 'double standard of mental health' which defined female psychiatric symptoms such as depression or frigidity as different from male psychiatric symptoms such as alcoholism and drug addiction or sociopathic personality. Chesler shows how psychology and psychiatry defined the gender bias within power relations inside the psychiatric institutions. Almost in a similar tone and within the context of psychiatry in England during 1830 to 1980, Elaine Showalter wrote *The Female Malady*.[14] She pointed out that since women outnumbered men in asylums, insanity was necessarily understood as a female malady. Although this view does not stand in case of the asylums of Bengal during the period, her argument that 'proper establishment of the menstrual function was viewed as essential to female mental health' holds true in defining female insanity in the asylums of Bengal.[15]

Nineteenth-century medical texts and reports on women's reproductive health in India often referred to frequent occurrences of puerperal mania and puerperal fever causing physical debility and

[12] Indrani Sen, 'The Memsahib's "Madness": The European Woman's Mental Health in Late Nineteenth Century India,' *Social Scientist* 33, nos 5–6 (May–June 2005): 26–48.

[13] Phyllis Chesler, *Women and Madness* (New York: Palgrave Macmillan, 2005).

[14] Elaine Showalter, *The Female Malady: Women, Madness, and English Culture, 1830–1980* (London: Virago, 1987).

[15] Showalter, *The Female Malady*, 56.

puerperal insanity among women. It was associated with a diverse form of mental illnesses linked to childbirth, which could affect women of any 'class'. In her work *Dangerous Motherhood*, Hilary Marland argued that 'puerperal insanity was very much a disorder that "belonged" to the nineteenth century in terms of its medical and social setting'.[16] There are several instances of this disorder listed in the nineteenth-century medical records of India. As physicians could not diagnose its causes precisely, they often referred to violent mania and severe melancholia among women, either during pregnancy, during childbirth, or within months of her delivery, as its symptoms. The asylum records do not contain any mention of puerperal insanity, although there were clear hints of symptoms similar to this disorder in the case histories written about the insane women in Bengal whenever the asylum doctors diagnosed any prenatal or postnatal woman's madness. Puerperal insanity was prevalent among patients admitted to asylums, but the absence of the term in nineteenth-century asylum records, despite its presence in reports on reproductive health, is debatable.

James Mills suggested that colonial asylums in India were meant to manipulate and regulate vagabonds and dangerous Indians and that in reality, asylums became areas of controversy and resistance to colonial rule. He pointed out that there were instances of lunatics who even within the confines of the asylums could make decisions and resist the regimes of discipline. Through a study of the intentions of the British behind establishing mental asylums in India, the way in which local people interacted with these establishments, and also from the records left behind by these institutions, he argued that his study does not 'accept the diagnosis of any of the convicts of the asylums of British India as sane'.[17] Mills pointed out that inmates often looked at mental hospitals as a place that they could use for their own ends. Therefore, these were not only places where families could put up the troublesome members of the household, but also, for the patients themselves, a place of shelter, work opportunities, and a refuge in times of personal crisis, in addition to viewing it as a place where they

---

[16] Hilary Marland, *Dangerous Motherhood: Insanity and Childbirth in Victorian Britain* (Basingstoke: Palgrave Macmillan, 2004), 4.

[17] Mills, *Madness, Cannabis and Colonialism*, 2.

might escape the rough discipline of prison regimes.[18] He studied psychiatry within the broader project of the colonial 'civilizing mission'. But his argument that the institutions of 'modern psychiatry' in India were beginning to be established in the period after 1858 is debatable as its line of descent could be drawn back from the early decades of the nineteenth century.

Houses of Madness analyses how definitions of insanity and various methods of treatment gradually developed even before the transfer of power from the East India Company to the Crown took place. It was in the asylums that definitions of insanity were forged, expanded, modified, corrected, and extended through experiments on the inmates of the asylum, both 'natives' and Europeans, and which finally paved the way for the emergence of psychiatry as a discipline in the late nineteenth century. Although there were certain restrictions on such practices for the patients at the European asylum, this study shows that as long as they were in the colonies they were not completely exempt from experiments at the hands of European physicians.

There have been several works by historians on the social history of medicine in colonial Bengal over the last few decades.[19] Waltraud Ernst's work is an important contribution in the field; her recent study on the 'lunatic asylums' of Bengal is very relevant to this work.[20] Nevertheless, areas like madness and mental asylums in colonial Bengal seem to have eluded most scholars.

---

[18] James Mills, 'The History of Modern Psychiatry in India 1858–1947,' *History of Psychiatry*, 12, no. 48, Part 4 (2001): 431–58.

[19] Poonam Bala, *Imperialism and Medicine in Bengal: A Socio-Historical Perspective* (New Delhi, Newbury Park, London: Sage Publications, 1991); Deepak Kumar and Raj Sekhar Basu (eds), *Medical Encounters in British India* (New Delhi: Oxford University Press, 2013); David Arnold, *The New Cambridge History of India: Science Technology and Medicine in Colonial India* (Cambridge: Cambridge University Press, 2008); Biswamoy Pati and Mark Harrison (eds), *The Social History of Health and Medicine in Colonial India* (London and New York: Routledge, 2009).

[20] Waltraud Ernst, 'Institutions, People and Power: Lunatic Asylums in Bengal, 1800–1900', in *The Social History of Health and Medicine in Colonial India*, edited by Biswamoy Pati and Mark Harrison (Oxford: Routledge, 2009), 129–50.

The present study on asylums is different from Erving Goffman's book *Asylums*[21] which is about 'total' institutions and not specifically about asylums, psychiatry, or psychology. By 'total institutions', he means places where inmates lived, worked, ate, slept, and lived a life separated from the outside world and within 'locked doors' and 'high walls'. These total institutions include tuberculosis sanitaria, mental hospitals, jails, concentration camps, and boarding schools, just to mention a few. My work also differs from Thomas S. Szasz's work. Szasz was a critic of the medicalization of mental illness. For him, mental illness is a social artefact with no scientific basis. In his book *The Manufacture of Madness*[22] he stated that institutional psychiatry was harmful to the so-called mental patient. This was not because it was liable to abuse, but rather because it harmed persons categorized as insane in its essential function. A person, according to him, was called deviant not only because his conduct differed from a socially observed norm, but because it also differed from a morally professed ideal. In *Myth of Mental Illness*,[23] he argued that mental illness was a social construct created by doctors, that is, mental illness was not a disease but a myth constructed by doctors. According to him, mental illnesses were no different from other diseases of the body. The sole difference was that while the former involves the head and was manifest through behavioural symptoms, the latter struck other organs and showed disruptive symptoms in that particular region of the body. He further mentions that what psychiatrists' term as mental illness is no more than a deviation from definitions of normative social behaviour. So, madness, as argued by Szasz, is a social and behavioural construct rather than a disease in itself. There is nothing called mental illness. It was a term which, according to him, outlived whatever benefits it might have had and functions only as a convenient 'myth'.

---

[21] Erving Goffman, *Asylums: Essays on the Social Situation of Mental Patients and Other Inmates* (New York: Anchor Books, 1961).

[22] Thomas S. Szasz, *The Manufacture of Madness: A Comparative Study of the Inquisition and the Mental Health Movement* (London: Routledge and Kegan Paul, 1971).

[23] Thomas S. Szasz, *The Myth of Mental Illness: Foundation of a Theory of Personal Conduct* (New York: HarperCollins Publications, 1974).

The term 'native' is used as the opposite of European. 'Natives', therefore, included all those 'lunatics' who were not admitted into the European Lunatic Asylum of Calcutta. The Bengal Presidency in the nineteenth century included Calcutta, Dacca, Bihar, and Orissa. This study is limited to the Lower Provinces because it was there that the European settlements were clustered during the period and where the major asylums were also located. Another reason for choosing Bengal as the area of study is because of the first European Lunatic Asylum of Calcutta. Following the establishment of Dacca and Moorshedabad Asylums in 1805 in the Lower Provinces of Bengal, many asylums were also gradually built in other parts of India. Therefore, it is necessary to know what was happening in the asylums of Bengal and what led to the establishment of asylums.

This book suggests an alternative way of looking at mental illness and its treatment in asylums. Through an understanding of the definitions of insanity as framed by the medical practitioners of the time, this study suggests that there is a correlation between definitions of insanity and its treatment with the construction of new asylum buildings and the spatial distribution within it. It shows how every aspect of treatment at the asylums was determined by the changing definitions of insanity, and both these aspects were directly associated with the construction and architecture of asylum buildings. Therefore, this book questions how far the medical supremacy that was established through various methods of treatment at the asylums helped the consolidation of the supremacy of the colonial rulers and also eventually stabilized their position in the field of medicine in nineteenth-century India.

Chapter 1, 'Madness and Madhouses of the Lower Provinces of Bengal', studies some of the 'native' asylums in Bengal and the European Asylum of Calcutta. What led to the establishment of these asylums? What factors determined the location of the site? How did the architecture of asylums reflect changes in the definitions of insanity? This chapter also explains how, among several other factors, the treatment of insanity determined the construction of buildings and different wards and cells within it. European patients sent from the districts were often admitted temporarily at the 'native' asylum before being shifted to the European Lunatic Asylum. Therefore, it also studies the kind of arrangements that were made for the patients at the European Asylum and if and how these differed during their temporary stay at the 'native' asylums. The physicians appointed at the asylums were not specially trained in the treatment of mental illness. Observations on insanity and asylums in Europe, in contrast, date back to the seventeenth century. Physicians in India largely derived their ideas from what was practised in Europe during the time. It is this process of implementation of the theory into practice that this chapter also looks at.

Chapter 2, 'The Treatment of the Insane: Conflict between Theory and Practice', discusses how through the application of different methods of treatment, the patients were taken care of in the asylums. In doing so, it raises certain questions on the issue: which method of treatment dominated the medical practices in the asylums and why was that so? What led to changes in the method of treatment over the nineteenth century? Was it possible to understand definitions of insanity in the nineteenth century without understanding the methods of treatment? Was there any correlation between these definitions and treatment? This chapter studies how the process of treatment changed over time from mechanical restraint to moral treatment through these questions. Medical treatment certainly played a significant role, but its practice lost significance during the mid-nineteenth century with the gradual dominance of moral treatment. By the end of the nineteenth century, however, medical treatment succeeded in regaining its dominance.

Chapter 3, 'Women in the Lunatic Asylums of Bengal', focuses on women diagnosed as 'lunatics'. What was their class composition? Why was it that the reasons for insanity in most of the women termed 'insane' remained 'unknown'? Was there anything specific to women's insanity that was different from the existing definitions of insanity? Was the understanding of insanity 'feminized' and were male and female insanity considered different? If so, were the methods of treatment different for males and females? This chapter thus looks at the definitions of 'mad' women located within the variegated definitions of insanity constructed by nineteenth-century physicians. Through this, it also seeks to answer why most cases of female insanity remained 'unknown' and how the 'unknown' cases were defined in the medical reports.

Chapter 4, 'The Role of Asylum Staff in the Treatment of Insanity', focuses on the members of the asylum staff. How and why did their role become significant in the daily functioning of the asylums? Did they play an important part in making decisions about daily activities in the asylums and of the patients? The asylum staff was appointed to treat patients with care and in a humane manner. Therefore this chapter makes an attempt to understand how far their method of dealing with patients really helped to cure the inmates.

MADNESS AND MADHOUSES OF THE LOWER PROVINCES OF BENGAL

THIS CHAPTER STUDIES THE DIVERSE definitions of madness that were formulated in the madhouses[1] of Bengal during the nineteenth century. It also seeks to understand whether those definitions of insanity when implemented into practice had any necessary impact on the shifts and changes related to the architecture of the asylums. Therefore, in order to delve further into the issue, it is likewise necessary to look into the geographic location of asylums (see Map 1.1); for instance, what kind of site and location was preferred and why that was so, and the external features of the asylums as well as its internal management.

INSANITY AND ITS DEFINITIONS

At every stage of their practice in the asylums in Bengal, European physicians not only followed the contemporaneous medical literature of England and Europe, but also tried to put it into practice. This transformation of practices ranged from the duties and qualifications of a superintendent to the changing perceptions, understandings, and

---

[1] The term 'madhouse' was often used in nineteenth-century England to refer to an asylum.

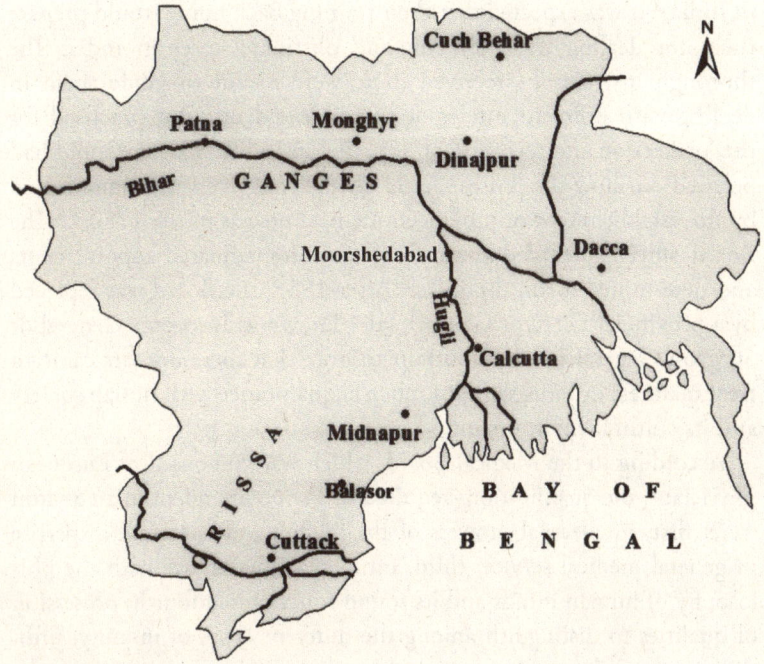

Map 1.1   Bengal Presidency during the Mid-nineteenth Century
Source: Author.
Note: Map not to scale.

definitions of insanity. They often made comparisons between the
asylums in Bengal and those in Europe and England. This got reflected
in the various definitions of insanity and the method of treatment for
the malady.

On completion of their medical training in Britain, medical
practitioners were sent to India to practice. In case the individual
was departing to join as a physician in one of the asylums in India,
then additional training from Bethlem, St. Luke's Hospital, or other
hospitals of a similar measure in England was considered all the more
necessary. If the doctor wanted to apply for the position of superintendent, he was required to receive training and experience as a
practitioner in any of asylums in India for a considerable period of time
before joining the office. The Medical Board considered this training
mandatory for 'judicious and skilful superintendence of lunatics'

in India.[2] It was expected that their training back home would prepare them for dealing with 'difficult and obstinate' cases in India. The thorough instructions received there were meant to guide them in dealing with different modes of coercion and restraint practised for the 'protection and recovery' of 'lunatics' in India.[3] David Arnold had pointed out how the 'bureaucratic' medical service was 'strengthened by the establishment of provincial medical boards in the 1780s'.[4] The Board officials included senior Surgeons who regulated appointments and determined medical policies. After 1857, the Board was replaced by a provincial Director General, later known as Inspector General or Surgeon General.[5] It is important to note that these doctors came to treat madness in India without much acquaintance with Indian society and its cultural environment.

According to the Medical Board, which was composed of European physicians, the qualifications required of a superintendent of an asylum were: first, intellectual prowess of the highest order; second, expertise in general medical service; third, intimate acquaintance with the philosophy of human minds and its sound functioning; fourth, possession of qualities to distinguish among the different types of insanity; fifth, skill to prescribe necessary remedies; sixth, judgement to direct the moral and physical regimen suited to each case; and finally, possession of sound discretion for the general management of the institution.[6] General Hospitals in India in the nineteenth century were considered by Lord Minto, the then Governor General of India, as the best schools for initiating and instructing medical servants on their arrival in India.

[2] Medical Board Proceedings, February 1811, An enclosure addressed to Lord Minto, Governor-General-in-Council, in a letter sent by R. Keys, Surgeon Presidency and Marine, to Robert Leny, Secretary Medical Board, dated 12 February 1811, National Archives of India, New Delhi [henceforth NAI].

[3] Medical Board Proceedings, Letter from R. Keys to Robert Leny, 12 February 1811.

[4] David Arnold, *The New Cambridge History of India: Science, Technology and Medicine in Colonial India* (Cambridge: Cambridge University Press, 2000), 58.

[5] Arnold, *The New Cambridge History of India*, 58.

[6] Medical Board Proceedings, July 1811, Letter sent to Mr Ricketts, Secretary to Government in the Public Department by Members of the Medical Board John Fleming, Walter Monro, I. G. Henderson, dated 15 July 1811, NAI.

Attendance at the hospitals was made compulsory. Lord Minto, on the advice of the Medical Board, directed all Surgeons on their arrival from Europe and Britain to practise under the Surgeon at the General Hospital for at least three months, following which they were appointed to the Sepoy Corps, Civil Stations, and often, even a battalion was exclusively entrusted to their charge.[7] The post of the Superintending Surgeon was of the highest rank in the medical department of Bengal Presidency.[8]

The officials of the Medical Board did not want asylum superintendents to change their locations from one asylum to another as the latter might lack the knowledge and expertise to deal with certain cases which might be specific to a particular asylum. This might materially impact upon the treatment and management of the insane.[9]

The Assistant Surgeon of an asylum, according to the Medical Board, was expected to have sufficient experience in order to prevent injuries that were often caused by patients. He was placed in charge of patients during the 'casual absence' of his superior or during the slack period when the nomination of a new superintendent was in process or until that officer became familiar with the cases under his charge. Usually, two Assistant Surgeons were appointed in an asylum according to their rank.[10]

The Magistrate had the discretionary power to send patients to the asylum. He not only had to consider complaints that were lodged against the Surgeon, but also had to guide him and issue orders whenever practicable. He sent a quarterly report on the conduct and accomplishment of the Surgeon to the committee in charge of the asylums and also reported to the government through the *sudder* about any neglect of his instructions. Any difference of opinion he had with the Surgeon had to be reported to this committee. The Surgeon received patients at the asylum only on the order of the Magistrate, Judges, or a committee

[7] Medical Board Proceedings, Letter from R. Keys to Robert Leny, 12 February 1811.

[8] Medical Board Proceedings, Number 40, 4 December 1817, Letter sent to Archibald Trotter, Secretary to Government in Public Department by Members of Medical Board, dated 4 December 1817, NAI.

[9] Medical Board Proceedings, Number 40, Letter from Members of the Medical Board to Archibald Trotter, 4 December 1817.

[10] Medical Board Proceedings, Number 40, Letter from Members of the Medical Board to Archibald Trotter, 4 December 1817.

formed for the purpose. They were, therefore, looked upon as judges of mental health while the Surgeon was merely a custodian acting on behalf of the Magistrate. The Surgeon could discharge certain cases from the hospital without consulting the Magistrate, but when the Magistrate wanted to discharge a patient against the opinion of the Surgeon, the case was referred to the Superintending Surgeon.[11] The Magistrate fixed the salaries of the asylum establishment and without his consent those could not be changed. A Surgeon was expected to know everything related to the treatment of insanity or else he was considered unfit for his job. But according to the Civil Assistant Surgeon of the Moorshedabad Asylum, a Surgeon often felt unhappy about having to work with a Judge, the committee, or the Magistrate and to see them as his superiors, as they had no knowledge required for the understanding and treatment of mental illness. The Magistrate who was endowed with the immediate power was usually junior in age to the Surgeon, but superior in terms of the rank held.[12] According to Section 4 of Act XXXVI of 1858, 'If the medical officer shall sign a certificate the form A in the schedule of this Act, and the magistrate shall be satisfied, on personal examination or other proof, that such person is a lunatic,'[13] an order of admission was issued. It also empowered Magistrates to severely punish any neglect or ill treatment of inmates who were sent back home from the asylums.[14]

The Inspector General of the Medical Department stated that a Surgeon deserved encouragement and support because he was completely

[11] Medical Board Proceedings, May 1842, Letter sent to W. Findon, Superintending Surgeon Presidency Division by A. Kean, Civil Assistant Surgeon, Moorshedabad, dated 26 March 1842, NAI.

[12] Medical Board Proceedings, Letter from A. Kean to W. Findon, 26 March 1842.

[13] Bengal Proceedings, Medical Department, Number 47, 27 February 1862, Letter sent to Officiating Junior Secretary to the Government of Bengal from A. Payne, Assistant Surgeon and Superintendent of the Asylums at the Presidency, dated 18 February 1862, Asia, Pacific and Africa Collections, British Library [henceforth APAC, BL].

[14] Bengal Proceedings, Medical Department, Number 10, 23 August 1862, Letter sent to A. Eden, Officiating Secretary to the Government of Bengal from J. McClelland, Officiating Principal Inspector General, Medical Department, dated 3 July 1862, APAC, BL.

responsible for the patients. This could be attained by bestowing on him the confidence of his employees and investing in him the power commensurate with his duties. The Surgeon was expected not to do any wrong either in regard to admission and discharge or in the treatment of the patients. In case of any wrong done, the Superintending Surgeon intervened. The overlapping jurisdiction of the Sudder Adalat with the Medical Board also increased the task of the Surgeon, who then had to forward monthly, half-yearly, and annual statements through the Magistrate. The right of visiting and inspecting the asylum continued to be held by the Sessions Judge who also had the right to communicate with the Superintending Surgeon when required.[15] The Judge disapproved of the prevailing medical system as it was not the one 'best calculated to draw out the best energies of the medical man'.[16]

The superintendents of asylums were regularly updated with news on insanity and its treatment in England and Europe. The Inspector General of Hospitals also approved of this. For instance, in 1862, the Superintendent Surgeon of Asylums in the Bengal Presidency requested the Secretary of State through the Inspector General of Hospitals to supply him regularly with copies of the Annual Reports of the Commissioners in Lunacy in England and Scotland, and of the Lunacy Inspectors in Ireland. In 1862, the Superintendent Surgeon of Bengal anxiously expressed that 'his office [was] at present entirely without information on the changes and improvements, which were made from time to time in Europe, in the internal management of asylums and the public official machinery by which the whole department was conducted and governed'.[17] According to him, such information was necessary at all times and particularly so when the government considered building a new asylum. The superintendents of asylums in the Presidency

[15] Bengal Proceedings, Medical Department, Number 10, Letter from J. McCelland to A. Eden, 3 July 1862.

[16] Medical Board Proceedings, Letter from A. Kean to W. Findon, 26 March 1842.

[17] General Proceedings, General Department, Number 58, April 1862, Letter sent to H. M. Macpherson, Principal Secretary Inspector General Medical Department by Arthur Payne, Assistant Superintending Surgeon of Asylums at the Presidency, dated 2 April 1862, West Bengal State Archives [henceforth WBSA].

were in charge of providing the necessary information regarding mental illness to the government. The then Superintendent Surgeon of Bengal referred to the psychological journals for references to medical understanding in England, although he considered it to be 'fragmentary and partial', and therefore, 'not valid for authoritative reference'.[18] Hence, for regular updates and detailed reports on asylums and mental illness in England, he officially applied to the Government of England to obtain copies of the Annual Reports of the Commissioners in Lunacy in England and Scotland and of the Lunacy Inspectors in Ireland.[19] The Inspector General of Hospitals considered it 'right' and 'necessary' for the Superintendents of Asylums to be acquainted with the current views and improvements in the management of the Insane in Europe.[20]

A comparison was frequently drawn by medical officers between the mortality of patients in the asylums in England and Bengal, although the social composition and condition in which patients were sent to the asylums in the two countries differed in many aspects. In the metropolitan and borough asylums of England, patients of the middle and pauper classes, with few exceptions, were admitted. It was punishable to keep a mentally ill patient in a private home in England without legal sanctions. In Bengal, according to James Wise, a very small proportion of 'lunatics' were admitted to asylums.[21] The Dacca District Superintendent's office recorded a total of 145 mentally ill persons who were maintained by their relatives at home.[22] Regarding this, the Superintendent of the Dacca Asylum stated that only those 'lunatics' who were criminals, or homeless, dangerous, or incurable, were admitted. Their illness often lasted for years, and it was only when the relatives were 'tired' of looking

[18] General Proceedings, General Department, Number 58, April 1862, Letter sent from Arthur Payne to H. M. Macpherson, 2 April 1862.

[19] General Proceedings, General Department, Number 58, April 1862, Letter sent from Arthur Payne to H. M. Macpherson, 2 April 1862.

[20] General Proceedings, Medical Department, Number 45, Letter from J. Forsyth to E. H. Lushington, 9 April 1862.

[21] James Wise, 'Report on the Dacca Lunatic Asylum for the Year 1871', in *Annual Report on the Lunatic Asylums of Bengal for the Year 1871* by J. Campbell Brown, Inspector General of Hospitals, Indian Medical Department (Calcutta: Bengal Secretariat Press, 1872), NAI.

[22] Wise, 'Report on the Dacca Lunatic Asylum', *Annual Report on the Lunatic Asylums of Bengal for the Year 1871*.

after them, or because their 'means were exhausted', that they admitted them to the asylums.[23]

This exemplified the medical officers' involvement with issues of insanity not only inside the asylums but outside them as well. By the 1870s, they were not only treating those who were admitted but also reaching out to those outside the asylums. A possible reason for this was that during the time, the asylum physicians were also recognized as the general physicians. More importantly, upper class families preferred that doctors visit at home instead of admitting their family members at an asylum in order to escape the shame and disgrace. Therefore, medical officers began treatment outside the asylum, took an initiative to reach out to the families of patients, and also kept a record of their post-treatment care once they were discharged from the asylum. For example, by 1894, the Superintendent of Dullunda Asylum was commended by the Government for his efforts in finding out the friends of 'harmless lunatics' and convincing them to take charge of the patients once they were discharged from the asylum.[24] The initiative taken by the medical officers was expected to open a scope for post-treatment observation of patients, while also help them to control the number of patients in asylums, thereby providing the chance to cure the maximum number of new cases. As the total number of inmates outgrew the space allotted to them, it became increasingly difficult for the officers to control the situation. The engagement of the asylum officers with the patients even after they were cured and discharged was reflected in the following lines by the Inspector General of Hospitals:

> It would be highly interesting could we ascertain what becomes of the discharged cured and relieved. Do these recovered and improved lunatics return to their occupations? How many die at their homes, and what time elapses between the dates of discharge and the fatal issue in each case?[25]

[23] Wise, 'Report on the Dacca Lunatic Asylum', *Annual Report on the Lunatic Asylums of Bengal for the Year 1871.*

[24] Home Department, Medical Board Proceedings, Number 78, July 1894, 'Report on the Lunatic Asylums of Bengal for the Year 1893,' by J. A. Bourdillon, Officiating Secretary to the Government of Bengal, NAI.

[25] Home, Medical, Number 100, September 1885, 'Report on the Lunatic Asylums of Bengal for 1884,' by J. Ware Edgar, Officiating Secretary to the Government of Bengal, NAI.

The Superintendent Surgeon of Bengal Presidency stated in 1862 that in the 'native' asylums 'unnecessary' admissions had become a common occurrence. The medical certificate was regarded as the only necessary evidence of mental illness, and patients suffering from temporary delirium, whether as a result of disease, debility, or intoxication, were transferred to the asylums. After a brief observation, he approved the admission of 'dangerous lunatics'. Admission of this category of patients was considered necessary for the safety of common people outside the asylum. Therefore, the majority of non-violent, non-dangerous inmates, according to him, should be treated in their own homes.[26]

By the 1870s, the Commissioners of Lunacy did not consider the information on the duration of insanity prior to admission as a necessary condition for admittance. Whenever a person in England became insane, he or she was given a certificate of insanity, and admitted to one of the numerous institutions existing across the country.[27] In England almost all 'lunatics' were under treatment, while in Bengal, as stated by J. Campbell, the great majority of them never reached the asylums. In most of the cases, the previous history was not known. Those sent in by the police were usually homeless people who were found wandering. The cause of mental illness among those was generally diagnosed as chronic.[28]

By 1872, the cause of mental illness could be attributed in only 20.6 per cent of the cases in the Dacca Lunatic Asylum. It was towards the end of the century that the asylum superintendents began to doubt the accuracy of the statements sent in by the police, although they had no other option but to rely on such statistics for necessary information. According to James Wise, the officials in England also faced similar difficulties in arriving at any conclusion regarding the cause of insanity amongst a large proportion of those admitted. He further said that Sir Charles Hood, in his 'Statistics of Insanity' stated that among 33.2 per cent of the cases admitted during the period between 1846 and 1855

[26] Bengal Proceedings, Number 47, Letter from A. Payne to Officiating Junior Secretary, 18 February 1862.

[27] Wise, 'Report on the Dacca Lunatic Asylum,' *Annual Report on the Lunatic Asylums of Bengal for the Year 1871.*

[28] Resolution, Judicial Department, 4 October 1872, *Annual Report on the Lunatic Asylums of Bengal for the Year 1871.*

to Bethlem, the reason for their madness could not be clearly ascertained. The fact that the causes of mental illness could not be determined amongst most of the patients at the time of admission in England made the job easier for the medical practitioners of Bengal. Therefore, Surgeon James Wise could very easily conclude:

> There is little wonder, therefore, that in Bengal we find it extremely difficult to indicate the cause which in each case excites or predisposes to insanity.[29]

Surgeon James Wise of Dacca commented on the prevalence and causes of insanity among different communities of eastern Bengal. Caste distinctions often signified differences in social customs and conditions, such as 'occupation, diet, mode of residence and life, habits, indulgences, and vices'. This, he believed, had a direct relation with the causes of insanity. Hence, without confining himself within the walls of the asylum, he looked into the surrounding localities for similar cases. But he was careful with his work as he knew that such investigations yielded useful and valuable results and helped in treating mental illness only when the examination was conducted with 'intelligence and care'. He believed this research would help medical officers understand the causes of insanity beyond the 'vague and other erroneous documents' that accompanied patients to the asylums. Dr Coates of Moydapore Asylum also had a similar impression. Thus, to get the right information regarding the causes of mental illness, the 'reception, habitual or incidental', of an unusually large number of patients from particular districts or localities, and variations in the forms of insanity taking place in different places[30] were beginning to be recorded.

J. Campbell was unwilling to accept the reason for an increase in admission from a particular district due to greater activity on the part of the Magistrate and the police.[31] Instead, he proposed that a true

[29] 'Report on the Dacca Lunatic Asylum for the Year 1872,' *Annual Report on the Lunatic Asylums of Bengal for the Year 1872*, by J. Campbell Brown, Inspector General of Hospitals, Indian Medical Department (Calcutta: Calcutta Press Company, 1873), NAI.

[30] 'Report on the Dacca Lunatic Asylum for the Year 1872,' *Annual Report on the Lunatic Asylums of Bengal for the Year 1872*.

[31] 'Report on the Dacca Lunatic Asylum for the Year 1872,' *Annual Report on the Lunatic Asylums of Bengal for the Year 1872*.

knowledge of the causation of insanity could only be obtained from a very careful investigation of particular cases with their antecedents, and an extensive knowledge of the social peculiarities, practices of individuals, and communities.[32] The 'native' of India, according to him, suffered more from intellectual than from emotional insanity, whereas the Europeans suffered from both 'intellectual and emotional' causes of insanity. Therefore, when an insane person in India suffered from delusions, as compared to Europeans, it was rarely considered to be 'violent or furious'. The initial stage of excitement subsided into a phase which was recorded as 'dull, stupid', and inactive. Unmoved by the intensity of their feelings when they lost control of their reasoning ability, European 'lunatics' often believed in themselves as 'great prophets, founders of religion, and conquerors of history'. The insane in India, under similar circumstances, also descended into a condition of 'intellectual prostration', which, according to medical reports, closely resembled the manifestations of dementia in Europe.[33] According to James Wise, it was possible that the apparent prevalence of insanity in one district as compared to another often depended on the instructions given to the police. Likewise, if a Magistrate insisted on all homeless 'lunatics' being sent into the sudder station, the proportion of patients from that particular district then exceeded those from an adjoining district where such an order was not enacted.[34] The massing of different categories of patients together often caused difficulties in their proper control and treatment, especially when limited space was a major cause of concern.[35]

By 1890, the College of Physicians issued their new 'nomenclatures' for classifying the different types of mental illness. The College stated that uniformity of classification would not be secured until some arbitrary definition of the various types of insanity was

---

[32] 'Report on the Dacca Lunatic Asylum for the Year 1872,' *Annual Report on the Lunatic Asylums of Bengal for the Year 1872.*

[33] Superintendent Surgeon R. Bird, 'Report on the Dullunda Lunatic Asylum,' *Annual Report on the Lunatic Asylums of Bengal for the Year 1872.*

[34] James Wise, 'Report on the Dacca Lunatic Asylum,' *Annual Report on the Lunatic Asylums of Bengal for the Year 1872.*

[35] Wise, 'Report on the Dacca Lunatic Asylum,' *Annual Report on the Lunatic Asylums of Bengal for the Year 1871.*

prescribed.[36] According to A. Hilson, the new nomenclature of mental diseases given by the College of Physicians in London was followed in the asylums of Bengal, but it had failed to secure uniformity of classification at the various asylums.[37] For instance, a considerable number of cases of 'toxic insanity' were known to have occurred in Patna, Dacca, Cuttack, and Berhampore, although there no such cases was registered at Dullunda. According to him, its absence at Dullunda could be accounted for by the difference of opinion held by the superintendents regarding the nature and cause of this particular form of insanity. Hence, A. Hilson stated that until medical officers of the College possessed any clear definition of the types of mental disease, it became impossible for them to have any approach to uniformity at the different asylums regarding 'toxic insanity'.[38]

Differences of categorization of insanity varied from one asylum to another, so accordingly, the statements in the annual returns of the asylums also differed. Thus, in some asylums, cases of acute mania which continued for months were transferred under the heading of chronic mania, whereas in another asylum, a year or more elapsed before this was done. In yet another instance, the original name remained unchanged through the entire period of a patient's residence in an asylum.[39]

On the question of the 'nomenclature' and the difficulties in the classification of some forms of mental diseases, the following note occurred in Dr Crombie's report:

Every year references are made to the uncertainty of nomenclature in the hands of different superintendents. As a matter of fact, there is room for difference

[36] Home, Medical, Number 133, July 1890, 'Resolution on Asylums of Bengal for the Year 1890,' by C. C. Stevens, Officiating Chief Secretary to the Government of Bengal, NAI.

[37] Home, Medical, Number 135, July 1890, 'Report on the Lunatic Asylums of Bengal for the Year 1889,' sent to the Chief Secretary to the Government of Bengal by A. Hilson, Inspector General of Civil Hospitals, Bengal, dated 8 April 1890, NAI.

[38] Home, Medical, Number 135, 'Report on the Lunatic Asylums of Bengal for the Year 1889,' 8 April 1890.

[39] 'Annual Report on the Lunatic Asylums of Bengal for the Year 1880,' sent to the Secretary to the Government of Bengal, Judicial, Political, and Appointment Departments by Arthur Payne, Surgeon General of Bengal, dated 28 March 1881, NAI.

of practice. The prevailing type of insanity in this part of India is that which is manifested by eccentricity, loquacity, and general joyfulness and absurdity of demeanour, generally without delusions and with no loss of intelligence.[40]

These cases, according to Crombie, fell under the division of chronic mania, as they showed 'exaltations of the emotional faculties'. While it was possible that a certain physician might classify it under chronic dementia, another, noticing the 'exaltation of emotion' would record it under chronic mania. The asylum physicians found it difficult to distinguish between melancholia and dementia, as in both the cases the patient showed similar symptoms: conveyed the same thought and disregard of surroundings, similar solitary habits, maintained silence or reluctance to speak, and did not maintain decency or personal cleanliness.[41] On the other hand, the distinction between dementia and imbecility was dependent on the case history. If the mental degradation, according to Crombie, occurred after the full development of the mental faculties, it became a case of dementia. If it was due to an arrested development of the mental powers in infancy, it was a case of imbecility.[42]

The 'descriptive rolls' based on which the diagnoses depended were considered 'worthless' by the asylum physicians, as they 'either contained no information whatever or were quite untrustworthy'.[43] The different types of mental illness were therefore not clearly defined. According to A. J. Cowie, the definitions 'dovetail, overlap, and merge' into one another, and as the case progressed, the identifications of the types of insanity often changed altogether. The diversity in the practice of some superintendents, according to the Inspector General of Hospitals in 1886, was chiefly due to a want of experience in the management and treatment of the patients. He further stated that accuracy, or an

[40] Home, Medical, Number 131, July 1886, 'Report on the Lunatic Asylums of Bengal for the Year 1885,' sent to the Secretary to the Government of Bengal, Medical and Municipal Department from A. J. Cowie, Inspector General of Civil Hospitals, dated 4 June 1886, NAI.

[41] Home, Medical, Number 131, 'Report on Lunatic Asylums of Bengal for the Year 1885,' 4 June 1886.

[42] Home, Medical, Number 131, 'Report on Lunatic Asylums of Bengal for the Year 1885,' 4 June 1886.

[43] Home, Medical, Number 131, 'Report on Lunatic Asylums of Bengal for the year 1885,' 4 June 1886.

approach to near accuracy came with a mature knowledge of and familiarity with the various forms and progress of mental diseases. Therefore, an important fallacy that occurred in the statistical records was the difficulty of separating first admissions from cases of recurrent insanity.[44]

The medical history sheet was considered useful by the physicians only when it was carefully filled up. But if carelessly prepared at the time of admission of the inmates, these documents were considered useless. During his inspection at the Dacca Lunatic Asylum in 1898, T. H. Hendeley observed that some of the certificates were incorrect. In several cases, men were described as being in good health when they were suffering from advanced phthisis. The Superintendent of the asylum pointed out that the medical history sheets, in many cases, provided very meagre and incomplete data and were returned for rectification. Therefore, the physicians wanted the medical history sheet to be carefully prepared by the officers who were responsible for the entries made in them. If the committing officers bestowed greater care and attention upon this part of their duty, many of the irregularities, the Inspector General believed, would disappear.[45]

A discussion on changes by the medical practitioners in the procedure of filling the medical sheets at the time of admission was not undertaken by the officers appointed for the task. Therefore, by 1900, of the total number of 220 patients admitted and readmitted during the year, 117 were criminals as against 78 in 1898, which, according to the Superintendent, was the largest number on record since 1880. These figures explained that the orders of the Government directing the exercise of a wise discretion in sending harmless patients whether criminal or non-criminal to asylums were not fully complied with. The Government, therefore, attempted to get the attention of the local authorities to the necessity of preparing these documents carefully.[46]

[44] Home, Medical, Number 131, 'Report on Lunatic Asylums of Bengal for the Year 1885,' 4 June 1886.

[45] *Annual Report on the Lunatic Asylums of Bengal for the Year 1898* by Colonel T. H. Hendeley, Inspector General of Civil Hospitals, Bengal (Calcutta: Bengal Secretariat Press, 1899), NAI.

[46] Home Department, Medical Branch, Number 52, September 1900, 'Annual Report on the Lunatic Asylums of India for 1899,' by E. N. Baker, Secretary to the Government of Bengal, NAI.

Since the asylum physicians endeavoured to achieve the best treatment for the patients through various experiments and observations, the system of 'infirm gang' was introduced at Dullunda and Dacca Asylums. According to the Inspector General of Hospitals,

> The infirm gang simply means that weakly looking persons are more frequently weighed, received some extra diet and are given tonics and drugs with the advantage of keeping off serious disease. It is a part of general management in an institution in which all the inmates are really diseased.[47]

Although the Government ordered the introduction of 'infirm gang' in all the asylums, the Superintendent of the Cuttack Asylum stated that the system was not necessary in that institution, as the number of sick patients was very small. The Superintendent of the Berhampore Lunatic Asylum also did not consider 'infirm gang' necessary, as, in his opinion, all deviations from normal condition, whether fits, excitement, paralysis, or other ailments, were to be closely observed by the Civil Hospital Assistant, and such cases kept in hospital wards or cells.[48] Judging, however, from the results obtained at Dacca, the Lieutenant Governor agreed with the opinion expressed by Colonel Hendeley that the system served to ward off serious diseases and that it would be given a through trial in all the asylums.[49]

Therefore, for several reasons, it was not easy to reach a particular definition of insanity, as various circumstances were closely associated with it. In the early nineteenth century there were not many discussions about the causes of insanity. Insanity was then defined as 'derangement of mind' without any further explanations. The treatment that followed was also very general, which focused mainly on the overall health of the inmates. Physical illnesses alone were taken into consideration. The initiative was taken to provide the patients with proper food and clothing along with several dosages of tonics to treat the problem. By the mid-nineteenth century, when insanity began to

[47] Home Department, Medical Branch, Number 52, 'Annual Report on the Lunatic Asylums of India for 1899,' by E. N. Baker.

[48] *Annual Report on the Lunatic Asylums of Bengal for the Year 1898*, by Colonel T. H. Hendeley.

[49] Home Department, Medical Branch, Number 52, 'Annual Report on the Lunatic Asylums of India for 1899,' by E. N. Baker.

be recognized as a disease, the situation got complicated. Several other factors gradually became part of the treatment of mental illness. One important factor was the question of space allotted to the inmates in the asylum. It became more and more necessary for the medical officers to segregate different categories of patients and treat them accordingly. Therefore, different types of rooms, such as dormitories, wards, and cells were constructed where patients suffering from similar kinds of illnesses were accommodated.

INCREASE IN ASYLUM POPULATION AND THE QUESTION OF MORTALITY

According to Surgeon J. Fullarton, the average number of cured patients discharged from all asylums of Bengal in 1876 was considerably lower than it was in former years. But, all the same, it compared favourably with the statistics of the public asylums of Middlesex and Surrey for the ten years from 1865 to 1874, compiled by the Lancet Commission on Lunatic Asylums. Considering the reduction in the proportion of recoveries in England, the Lancet Commission stated:

> The inference is, we think, unfavourable to the class of cases sent to asylums rather than to the repute of the system of treatment pursued. The policy of finding accommodation for '*all* the lunatics in the country' creates a miscellaneous crowd, of which comparatively a small proportion can be considered susceptible of cure or radical improvement.[50]

The Surgeon General quoted these lines from *Lancet*, the chief medical journal of England during the time, as he considered the same reason to be equally applicable in case of Bengal.[51]

Statistics in Europe showed that changes in seasons had some influence on mental illness. Consequently, the Superintendent of the Patna

[50] *Annual Report on the Insane Asylums of Bengal for the Year 1876*, by J. Fullarton Beatson, Surgeon General, Indian Medical Department to Secretary to the Government of Bengal Judicial Department, Fort William, 16 July 1877 (Calcutta: Bengal Secretariat Press, 1877), NAI.

[51] *Annual Report on the Insane Asylums of Bengal for the Year 1876*, by J. Fullarton Beatson.

Lunatic Asylum concluded that summer saw a larger ratio of admissions into the asylum. According to him, at certain times of the year, this steady increase of population into the Patna Asylum as well as into other asylums required the attention of the government.[52]

On several occasions, asylum superintendents of Bengal ascribed different reasons for the increase and decrease in population in the asylums. Incidents of readmission were often considered as one of the reasons for such an increase. For instance, a woman who was returned to her mother after treatment at the Dacca Asylum was readmitted to the asylum after two years. She was found wandering on the street and 'picked up' by the police. During her second visit to the asylum, she was registered as a patient with dementia. According to the doctors the reason for her dementia was epilepsy.[53] According to Dr Bird of the Bhawanipore Lunatic Asylum, mental illness, like other diseases, was liable to fluctuate. Dr Wise of the Dacca Asylum found it difficult to account for an increase in madness in 1872, and he presumed that the dengue epidemic during the year might have had some influence, though he also noted that the excess patients came from those districts of Bengal where cases of dengue were not registered. Dr Simpson of the Patna Lunatic Asylum was inclined to attribute the circumstances to 'heated climate'. Dr Coates of the Moydapore Asylum attributed the increase to a greater activity on the part of the police. But according to Inspector General J. Campbell, it was difficult to determine how far an 'increased production of the disease or increase of vigilance and vigour by police' accounted for the increase in the number of 'lunatics' in 1872.[54] Rather, he pointed out that the fluctuation in admission was often due to 'aetiological' and administrative factors.

The Annual Report of 1872 showed that the largest number of patients were admitted during the rainy season: 62 per cent of the annual admissions of that year were admitted between April and September.

[52] Superintendent B. Simpson, 'Report on the Patna Lunatic Asylum,' *Annual Report on the Lunatic Asylums of Bengal for the Year 1872.*

[53] Wise, 'Report on the Dacca Lunatic Asylum', in *Annual Report on the Lunatic Asylums of Bengal for the Year 1872,*

[54] *Annual Report on the Lunatic Asylums of Bengal for the Year 1872*, by J. Campbell Brown.

But there were disagreements amongst asylum superintendents on this issue as well. Some would consider excess 'heat' while others would cite an excess of 'rain' as the reason for an increase in admission. According to Dr Simpson, a greater number of admissions took place during summer; 'heat', he argued, could be the reason for the variance in the larger number of admissions in one year as compared with another. Dr Wise noticed the same circumstance, but in his report for 1871 he attributed the increase in number of admissions to the rains. This was because 'lunatics' from several districts often reached the Dacca Asylum by boats, which was a convenient mode of travel in these regions as the place was well-connected with rivers. Such instances, although applicable in case of Dacca according to the Inspector General, was not at all relevant for Bihar where people usually travelled on land.[55]

The decrease in lunacy was therefore explained by the reduction in the 'admissions under the head of acute mania' and 'uncertainty of nomenclature in the hands of different Superintendents', and 'changes in the Superintendent of Asylums', affected the nomenclature of diseases.[56] A medical officer entered his acute or chronic mania patients under the category of melancholia. The longer the chronic cases were retained in the asylums, the lower was the rate of recoveries. Again, a certain number of criminal patients were frequently admitted to the asylum, and those, along with records of non-criminal patients, produced mixed statistics of the asylums. Hence, the Inspector General of Hospitals stated that the identification of different types of insanity and their interpretations during admission was the usual practice in British, American, and continental Asylums. J. Campbell's explanation for overcrowding in the asylum was quite dissimilar from other medical practitioners. 'Native' insanity, according to him, was less 'expressive' in comparison to that of Europeans. Therefore the medical officers in India could not reach a conclusion on how long it would need for a patient to recover. Even when treated over a long period of time, the progress of treatment was not always discernible unless

[55] *Annual Report on the Lunatic Asylums of Bengal for the Year 1872*, by J. Campbell Brown.
[56] Home, Medical, Number 131, 'Report on Lunatic Asylums of Bengal for the Year 1885,' 4 June 1886.

carefully observed. Therefore, according to him, overcrowding was often due to cured patients staying on in the asylum 'unnoticed by the Superintendent'. To guard against such an oversight, the practice of conducting a rigid mental examination on each of the patients was implemented on a monthly basis.[57]

By the 1870s, the Government had altered the rules of admission to asylums. Payment was made compulsory for every patient.[58] This was done to reduce the number of admissions to the asylums while at the same time cure the maximum number of patients already admitted. This was necessary to maintain the number of admissions within the restricted space and within a limited number of asylums. This, the Superintendent of the Patna Asylum thought, would help to reduce the number of admissions. At the same time, judging from numerous complaints, he observed that the measure seemed a most unpopular one. He was apprehensive that such measures would induce people to confine and ill-treat their insane relatives at home, in order to prevent their falling into the hands of the police and also being sent to an asylum where they would have to pay for their maintenance.[59] The imposition of a fixed payment for every patient helped the government to control new admissions. That the government's rules for payment for every individual faced criticism was reflected in a report of a native newspaper of Bengal. It stated that as the lowest rate for detaining patients was fixed at Rs 12 a month, it would be beyond the ability of the poor to admit patients to the asylum. The newspaper appreciated the decision of the government to arrest all 'lunatics' found wandering on the streets. But it also pointed out that the government should not only detain those non-violent, poor 'lunatics' who were found wandering but also those who behaved in an 'unruly' manner in their own homes.[60]

[57] Surgeon R. Bird, 'Report on the Dullunda Lunatic Asylum,' *Annual Report on the Lunatic Asylums of Bengal for the Year 1872.*

[58] Simpson, 'Report on the Patna Lunatic Asylum,' *Annual Report on the Lunatic Asylums of Bengal for the Year 1872.*

[59] Simpson, 'Report on the Patna Lunatic Asylum,' *Annual Report on the Lunatic Asylums of Bengal for the Year 1872.*

[60] *Dainik o Samachar Chandrika*, 3 April 1894, Native Newspaper Reports of Bengal, 1894, NAI.

According to A. Payne, Superintendent of Dullunda Asylum, admissions of patients could finally be controlled in asylums only after the implementation of strict rules for payment as well as instructions given to Magistrates to send only 'specialized classes of lunatics'. Since the promulgation of the Order, the Government of Bengal took formal notice of some prevailing irregularities with regard to transmission, thereby substantially reducing the number of persons admitted at Dullunda. Most of the cases admitted by the 1870s at Dullunda included both criminal and chronic cases.[61] He further stated that in India, unlike in England, the reluctance to speak of 'hereditary tendencies' and 'disclose the habits' that hinted at the initial stage of the occurrence of mental illness often led to errors in mistaking the first symptoms of the disease as its causes. This was mainly noticed among patients from poor financial backgrounds, amongst whom the information regarding the cause of mental illness was often not procured unless the person was suffering due to the consumption of intoxicating substances, for instance, smoking *ganja* (cannabis). Under such circumstances, a probable cause of the illness was often recorded in the descriptive rolls.[62]

But the rules for payment also could not solve the problem of increase in asylum population towards the end of the nineteenth century. Both the Magistrate and the police were criticized by medical officers and held responsible for the increase in the number of inmates in the asylums. In order to get rid of 'troublesome' persons, police officers found it easy to introduce the word 'dangerous' into the short history of a case—describing a particular act or tendency of a person as such—which they then presented to the Magistrate. The Superintendent of Dullunda Asylum, A. Payne, anticipated that unless restricted or criticized by the Magistrate, this would be done to a greater extent and more freely. Hence, by 1885, the Government of India ordered only those patients who required care or restraint, and who might be reasonably anticipated to improve under treatment, to be admitted to mental hospitals, while

[61] 'Report on the Dullunda Asylum for the Year 1876,' by Superintendent A. J. Payne *Annual Report on the Insane Asylums of Bengal for the Year 1876*.

[62] *Annual Report on the Lunatic Asylums of Bengal for the Year 1879* by A. Payne, Surgeon General Bengal (Calcutta: Bengal Secretariat Press, 1880), NAI.

those diagnosed as partially insane as well as those seen as 'harmless' patients were to be kept out of them.[63]

ON ASYLUMS

It is within this context that both the geographical locations and the question of spatial distribution both inside and outside the asylums of Bengal are dealt with. Any discussion on the proposition of a new asylum always included the question of location, the plan of the asylum, and the inner and outer design of the building. The major asylums in the Lower Provinces of Bengal, which functioned throughout the nineteenth century included Dullunda, Dacca, Patna, Cuttack, and Berhampore, and the Bhawanipore Lunatic Asylum, particularly for the Europeans. While insanity and its treatment were a cause of concern, questions related to the construction of asylums, its location, and the question of spatial distribution was also taken equally into consideration by the medical officers. Amongst several asylums established in Bengal during the period, there was only one European asylum in Calcutta and the remaining were all 'native' ones. Both the European and 'native' asylums were maintained by the government, other than the establishment of a private European asylum, which functioned for a very short period of time in Calcutta. The European asylum was built to temporarily detain European 'lunatics' before they were shipped back to England for further treatment. The asylums at Moorshedabad and Hazareebagh functioned for a very short time. Inmates from those asylums were gradually shifted to Dullunda, Dacca, and Berhampore asylums.

EUROPEAN LUNATIC ASYLUM

The European Insane Hospital in Calcutta (see Map 1.2) was the oldest asylum and could be dated back to the 1780s. Its social composition was limited to European military personnel as initially this institution was primarily concerned with the treatment of the physically and

[63] Home, Medical, Number 102, September 1885, Letter sent to the Secretary to the Government of Bengal, Municipal, Medical Department, from A. Mackenzie, Secretary to the Government of India, dated 19 September 1885, NAI.

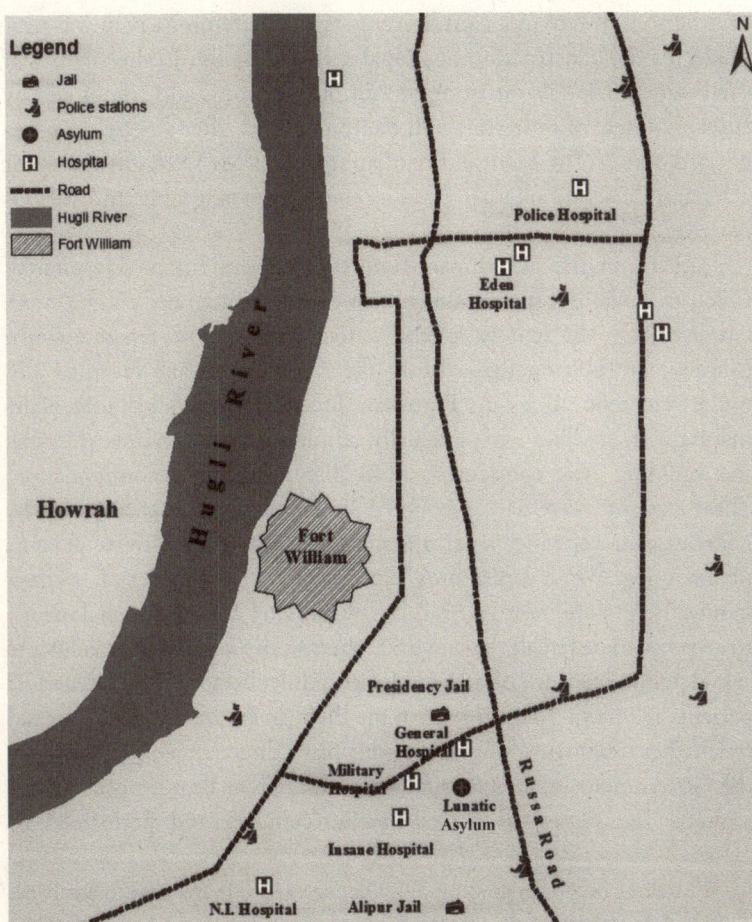

Map 1.2   Calcutta, 1893
Source: Author.
Note: Map not to scale.

mentally unfit soldiers. The asylum, therefore, continued to be under the supervision of the Military Department until its social composition changed, following which the General Department took charge. Among the physically and mentally unfit, it was difficult to control the 'troublesome' patients, especially those who were also considered as the 'most furious maniacs'. Such inmates were categorized as 'noisy' and 'outrageous' as they were known to hinder the 'perfect recovery of others who were in a convalescent state'. Therefore, a plan was proposed for the construction of a separate building but in the vicinity of the Insane Hospital consisting of four or five rooms and a floor laid by *chunar* stones, in order to avoid dampness even after frequent washes of the floors.[64] The Medical Board approved of Mr Dick's proposal for a separate accommodation for the 'more unmanageable and furious patients'.[65]

Initially, in the government-funded European Insane Hospital of Calcutta, only Europeans along with very few 'vagrant natives' were admitted. On the removal of the 'native' patients to a separate establishment in 1805 on Russa Road, the European Insane Hospital also underwent renovations. As European 'lunatics' who could individually maintain themselves were gradually admitted to the Insane Hospital, the building was considered unsuitable for their accommodation. These patients were accommodated in a new private asylum run by Mr. Beardsmore, which was constructed in 1818. The private patients placed under Mr. Beardsmore's supervision were maintained by their family, friends, and relatives.[66] This new building was constructed mainly to accommodate female patients and others whose families were willing to 'avoid public exposure' of such a 'misfortune'. It also accommodated those patients whose families did not want them to be removed to England for further treatment.[67] Following this plan, three female patients from the Government Insane Hospital were admitted at Beardsmore's private asylum. The periodical duties were undertaken and performed by

[64] Medical Board Proceedings, 27 October 1796, Letter sent to the President and Members of the Hospital Board from Mr Dick, Surgeon to the Hospital for Insane, Calcutta, dated 15 October 1796, NAI.

[65] Medical Board Proceedings, Letter sent to G. M. Barlow, Secretary to Government from A. Campbell, Secretary Medical Board, dated 17 October 1796, NAI.

[66] General Proceedings, General Department, Number 15, 18 May 1836, Letter sent to George Auckland, Governor General of India in Council by Beardsmore, Superintendent of the Private Lunatic Asylum, dated 5 May 1836, WBSA.

[67] Medical Board Proceedings, Number 14, 13 January 1821, Enclosure attached to a letter sent to W. Ogilvy, President and Member of the Medical Board from Charles Lushington, Secretary to Government in General Department, Council Chamber, dated 15 December 1820, NAI.

Mr Robinson and the internal management was left entirely in the care of Beardsmore who was also assisted by his wife, Mrs Beardsmore. The profits derived from the treatment were equally divided amongst the three of them.[68] The rules and regulations for admission of private and public patients at Beardsmore's asylum varied.[69] A detail of the asylum rules and regulations is given in Appendices I, II, and III.

The Board was anxious about finding a suitable accommodation for the European inmates of both the private and public hospitals. The asylum officers were not very content with Mr Beardsmore's private asylum. Hence, they adopted necessary measures to select the most suitable place for the construction of an asylum for the 'comfortable reception' of Europeans.

After a long search, the Medical Board officials, along with the Mr Robinson, chose a house lying in the rear of the Jaun Bazaar in central Calcutta. The house was located to the northeast of the Persian Office of the Company. The Board approved the condition of the house as appropriate because the building was spacious and placed in the midst of a large open area at a considerable distance from a public road, and sufficiently open for access to air from every quarter. It was regarded as perfectly suited to carry out the regulations meant for the asylum and also to avert the chances of irritation caused to the patients from the external environment. Since it was situated in the vicinity of several houses inhabited by 'respectable families', the Board officials were apprehensive that it might be a cause of public nuisance if it was converted into a 'madhouse'. However, the officials appealed for the government's consent. The government 'seriously' objected to the selection of the Board. The Governor-General-in-Council ordered the Board to select a suitable premise in the more solitary parts of the city or in its environs.[70] Thereafter, Mr Robinson selected another house occupied by one Mr Futton at Chowringhee. Although the Board approved of necessary

[68] Medical Board Proceedings, Number 14, Enclosure in Letter from Charles Lushington to W. Ogilvy, 15 December 1820.

[69] Medical Board Proceedings, Number 14, Enclosure in Letter from Charles Lushington to W. Ogilvy, 15 December 1820.

[70] Medical Board Proceedings, Number 26, 13 April 1819, Letter sent to W. Ogilvy, President and Member, Medical Board from C. Lushington, Secretary to Government in General Department, dated 30 March 1819, NAI.

additions that Robinson proposed for the building, they still did not think it suitable for accommodating European patients.[71] Therefore, that building was also rejected. Robinson died in 1819 and Mr Sawers became the next superintendent of the old Insane Hospital maintained by the government. He was put under constant pressure by the Board to find a suitable accommodation for the European patients. He objected to the Board's proposal to keep them in the private dwelling maintained by Beardsmore. This, according to him, could have proved a 'nuisance' for those in the neighbourhood, particularly because the ground floor rooms of a common dwelling house would not allow enough space for the patients being divided into classes according to the degree of malady or their status in society. Along with that, the small area was considered unsuitable for the free circulation of air necessary for the well-being of the patients. Another cause of worry for the officials was that the rooms were very closely placed, which was not conducive to housing 'quiet' patients in the same space as the 'noisy and mischievous' ones. Under such conditions, he approved of the Board's proposal for the design of a new construction.

In the new building, eleven rooms, each 20-feet long both on the ground and on the first floor that would run parallel to each other with a large door at both ends, were proposed. This was considered ideal as it would not only provide free circulation of air, but the rooms were also designed in a way that ensured that inmates in one room would not disturb those in another. A 15-feet-wide veranda along the entire length of the building, was proposed for the southeast side. On the northwest side, there was to be no veranda as that would have left the room hot during the summer and cold in the winter. Hence, a veranda with venetian blinds was added to the whole length of the northwest side, and a wall made on each veranda dividing the house into four distinct sections. This division was meant to allow the segregation of the patients into classes according to their positions in society as well as their degree of malady.

The private asylum initially established by the late Mr Robinson was considered a great advantage to the community, because the terms of

[71] Medical Board Proceedings, Number 28, 13 April 1819, Letter sent to James Jameson, Secretary, Medical Board from Mr Robinson, Superintendent for the House of Reception for the European Insane, dated 20 March 1819, NAI.

the asylum were not rigid; rather, they were relevant to the condition of the patient. The building in which the public patients were eventually accommodated were formerly occupied by female inmates. Hence, the interior was restructured; a dividing wall and separate rooms were made to accommodate public patients.[72] The Board was apprehensive of mentally ill patients residing in a private house and was, therefore, prompt in establishing a separate building in a secluded area maintained by the government. The officials were anxious that the superintendent of a private asylum living in his own quarters might not be as dutiful as he would be expected to be, as he was not only expected to be present in the midst of his patients, regardless of their malady or their former official rank, but also to sacrifice and remain detached from all the comforts of a family life.[73]

Due to the unavailability of any 'proper' accommodation, the Board finally decided to continue the admission of patients to the old Insane Hospital with certain renovations and additions to the building. They corresponded to Mr Sawers' proposal for the extension of the veranda and the construction of a wall.

According to the new plan proposed by the Board, a wall was constructed in the centre of the building with a door and a staircase to the west. The wall was meant to divide the interior into four separate compartments and allow further classification of patients according to their 'rank in life and kind or degree of sanity'.[74] The lower room of the house on the east was arranged for the admission of female patients. It was separated from the men's quarters by a partition wall, and was elevated well above the ground to avoid damp.[75] Initially rooms allotted for women in the private asylum were 'damp, gloomy

[72] Medical Board Proceedings, Number 35, 24 August 1819, Letter sent to James Jameson, Secretary, Medical Board from Mr Sawers, Surgeon, Insane Hospital, dated 22 August 1819, NAI.

[73] Medical Board Proceedings, Number 16, 9 October 1819, Letter sent to C. Lushington, Secretary to Government in General Department by James Jameson, Secretary Medical Board, dated 21 September 1819, NAI.

[74] Medical Board Proceedings, Number 16, Letter from James Jameson to C. Lushington, 21 September 1819.

[75] Medical Board Proceedings, Number 16, Letter from James Jameson to C. Lushington, 21 September 1819.

and sultry' and 'surrounded by trees'. Gradually, with an increase in the number of women in general and those of upper-class women in particular, internal arrangements were restructured. Hence, the officials decided to shift female patients to the top floor of the 'dry and airy' building that was formerly occupied by men.[76] Male inmates of the asylum, most of whom were soldiers, were given the first preference during their admission. They were always allotted better rooms than women.

The Board's observations regarding the European inmates of the lower classes at the Government Insane Hospital for Europeans was almost similar to its observations about lower-class 'natives'. Interestingly, the Victorian notion of class was reflected in the decision of the European physicians so far that it almost put the 'native' and European inmates of lower ranks on the same footing, blurring the boundaries of race and class. According to James Jameson, Secretary, Medical Board,

> the inmates of the Insane Hospital at this place are generally individuals taken from the lower classes of society, none of whom at any time enjoyed the luxuries and comforts usually possessed by persons in the better ranks of life. To such individuals while under confinement all that are requisite by way of maintenance is that they should be treated with the humanity and kindness due to their deplorable condition. They are not from education or habit fitted to enjoy pleasures or distinction of a higher sort and to give them a set at the table of the surgeon and show them the attention and difference usually paid to persons in the rank of gentlemen would probably rather tend further to unhinge their minds than to lessen their malady. This remark is peculiarly applicable to the patients in the hospital, not one of whom is of better condition than that of the soldier in the rank. It almost involves an absurdity to suppose that the medical officers should associate with such persons and hold with them any further intercourse than with [what] is absolutely necessary towards the faithful discharge of his purely professional duties.[77]

[76] Home Department, Medical Proceedings, Number 16, 9 October, 1819, Letter sent to C. Lushington, Secretary to the Government, General Department from James Jameson, Secretary Medical Board, Medical Board Office, dated 21 September 1819, NAI.

[77] Home Department, Medical Board Proceedings, Number 16, Letter from James Jameson to C. Lushington, 21 September 1819.

This exemplified that the Board did not even want the Superintendent to get too involved with the inmates of the lower ranks as they were worried that too much association with them might hinder their healing regimen. This professional position of the caretakers of the mentally ill therefore marked a deviation in the method of treatment with the process of segregation, and often led the officers to overlook the treatment of patients. But the position of the inmates was considerably better off in the 'native' asylums, where in the absence of class segregation, the methodology of treatment was simpler.

Finally, the government extended the lease of the old Insane Asylum for another ten years.[78] The asylum was visited by the Magistrate and the members of the Medical Board. The former appreciated the condition of the asylum mainly because of its construction in a dry and airy location. But he also recommended the provision of a commode and a chamber pot in each of the wards in addition to other indispensible articles necessary for health and cleanliness.[79] This was unlike the situation in the 'native' asylums where provisions for a toilet inside the wards were thought of as a necessity by the medical officers at a much later date.

The Government made a proposal to the Medical Board suggesting temporary accommodation of the European patients of the Insane Hospital either at the 'native' Hospital of Calcutta or at the General Hospital. The Medical Board inspected both the hospitals and firmly refused the proposal. This was not only because Europeans were sent back home at the earliest for their further recovery, but because the coexistence of mentally ill Europeans and 'natives' was unacceptable to the colonial rulers. Moreover, the 'native' Insane Hospital, which the Board had built to accommodate 'native' patients, was thought unfit for the reception of the Europeans. The Board further stated that not only was the 'native' Insane Hospital full of patients from the lower classes, it also did not have the conveniences or 'roominess', which, was necessary for

[78] Medical Board Proceedings, Number 18, 6 November 1819, Letter sent to James Jameson, Secretary Medical Board from C. Lushington, Secretary to Government in General Department, dated 6 November 1819, NAI.

[79] Medical Board Proceedings, Number 18, 6 November 1819, Enclosure attached to a letter sent to C. Lushington, Secretary to Government in General Department from H. Shakespear, Officiating Chief Magistrate, dated 6 November 1819, NAI.

the recovery of the European patients in a hot climate.[80] The central location of this asylum near the General Hospital showed that it was located on sites similar to that of other hospitals and public buildings within close proximity of a city or town. 'Native' asylums were also built in a central location during the early nineteenth century. But those gradually shifted to the outskirts, as moral treatment gained its significance by the mid-nineteenth century. By the end of the nineteenth century, asylums again became a part of the central locations of a town or city. This shift in asylum location was determined by a change in understanding insanity as a disease, which could be medically cared for.[81]

Another cause of worry, which prevented the Medical Board from admitting the patients at the Insane Hospital, Calcutta, was that the residence of the medical officer was at a distance from the hospital. This, according to them, would deprive the European patients of constant attention, which was necessary for their recovery.[82] The Board also did not want to admit European patients at the General Hospital because

> the admission of madmen who from the nature of their malady are continually liable to be noisy and refractory among patients to suffering under common disorders would certainly be very objectionable. So strange a mixture would prove prejudicial to the generality of the patients and might perhaps in the end be injurious to the character of the institution.[83]

The Honourable Court of Directors gave instructions in 1821 to abandon the Insane Hospital under the impression that the public insane patients would be maintained at a cheaper rate in England and the climate there would also prove far more conducive to their recovery. It was also decided that during the short period of their stay they would not be detained at the 'native' Insane Hospital. Therefore,

[80] Medical Board Proceedings, Number 14, 5 February 1821, Letter sent to C. Lushington, Secretary to Government in General Department from James Jameson, Secretary Medical Board, dated 5 February 1821, NAI.

[81] This is discussed in more detail in Chapter 2.

[82] Medical Board Proceedings, 5 February 1821, Letter from James Jameson to C. Lushington, 5 February 1821.

[83] Medical Board Proceedings, 5 February 1821, Letter from James Jameson to C. Lushington, 5 February 1821.

the government entered into a contract with Mr Beardsmore, who was known for his 'humanity, temper and prudence in the treatment and custody of insane persons at his Asylum'.[84] The Medical Board considered him fit and worthy of being trusted with the very delicate and responsible charge of persons labouring under mental illness.[85] Prior to his opening of the private institution, Mr Beardsmore was associated with the European Insane Hospital for five or six years and was entrusted as a subordinate officer who was responsible for the management of the patients.[86]

The public patients were housed temporarily at his private asylum, also known as the House of Reception, at the rate of Rs 100 per month for those of the upper class and Rs 50 per month for those of the lower class.[87] Within that fixed amount, Beardsmore was responsible for their safe custody, as well as clean and comfortable accommodation. He also supplied them with shoes, bedding, clothing, necessary medication, and food.[88]

Anglo-Indians of different 'denomination, without reference to colour or rank in life' were admitted at Beardsmore's private asylum by the authority of the members of the Medical Board and the Chief Magistrate of Calcutta. They had been previously admitted at the Insane Hospital.[89] People accommodated as first class patients usually got single rooms. But, meals were taken together at the public table

[84] Medical Board Proceedings, Number 5, 24 February 1821, Letter sent to W. Ogilvy, President and Member, Medical Board from C. Lushington, Secretary to Government in General Department, dated 20 February 1821, NAI.

[85] Medical Board Proceedings, Number 2, 5 March 1821, Letter sent to J. Adam, Assistant Surgeon from James Jameson, Secretary, Medical Board, dated 26 January 1821, NAI.

[86] Medical Board Proceedings, Number 3, 5 March 1821, Letter sent to James Jameson, Secretary, Medical Board from Mr Adams, Assistant Surgeon, dated 28 February 1821, NAI.

[87] Medical Board Proceedings, Number 10, 19 February 1821, Letter sent to James Jameson, Secretary, Medical Board from Beardsmore Superintendent Private Lunatic Asylum, dated 15 February 1821, NAI.

[88] Medical Board Proceedings, Number 10, Letter from Beardsmore to James Jameson, 15 February 1821.

[89] General Proceedings, General Department, Number 15, Letter from Beardsmore to George Auckland, 5 May 1836.

along with patients of lower classes. Violent or refractory inmates were maintained in a separate building within the compound, which was well-lit, ventilated, and had a large veranda for physical exercise. Meals were sent to them from the public table. Beardsmore claimed that they were given the 'best quality food from the market'. While the quality of food remained the same, the menu differed. The dishes for the first-class patients were dressed in a more savoury manner and included ducks, fowl, and fish, occasionally along with the various seasonal fruits as well as puddings, tarts, jellies, and cheese. The members of the Medical Board who occasionally visited the asylum during the hours of meal expressed their satisfaction with the liberal treatment given to the patients. The attire of upper-class patients was taken care of in accordance with their social status. Convalescent patients of higher rank were encouraged to spend the daytime in the upstairs area of the asylum with Mr Beardmore and his family. Within the personal space of Beardsmore's accommodation they were encouraged to read newspapers, books, and engage in *rational* conversations with the proprietor and his family. According to Mr Beardsmore all this was done 'to induce the unfortunate individuals to forget as far as practicable the condition in which they are accidentally placed'.[90]

In 1853, Mrs Sims, the new proprietor of the asylum, stated that amongst the public patients of the insane hospital, a few had recently become insane. The great majority of the cases were usually treated in regimental and other hospitals scattered all over India. Eventually, they were admitted at the lunatic asylum to be shipped back to Europe.[91] This was done indiscriminately without reference to the probability of recovery in the asylum or otherwise.[92] Of the Europeans who continued

[90] General Proceedings, General Department, Number 15, 9 November 1836, Letter sent to H. J. Prinsep, Secretary to Government in General Department from Mr Beardsmore, Proprietor and Superintendent, Bhawanipore Lunatic Asylum, dated 18 October 1836, WBSA.

[91] Medical Board Proceedings, Number 53, 15 February 1853, Letter sent to K. Mackinon, Secretary, Medical Board from Mrs Sims, Proprietor, Bhawanipore Lunatic Asylum, dated 12 February 1853, NAI.

[92] Medical Board Proceedings, Number 53, Letter from Mrs Sims to K. Mackinon, 12 February 1853.

to live at the asylum during 1853, one was found wandering about in the bazaars of Calcutta for months and was brought back to the house by the police. Another European was treated for mental illness at the Regimental Hospital and then sent to the asylum in July 1849. A woman, whose husband was stationed in the 80th regiment, was also found wandering on the streets. She was diagnosed with insanity and treated at Regimental Hospital before being shipped to Calcutta. Another European woman was also cured.[93] These instances showed that it was not only 'native' patients who were picked up from the street and admitted into the asylums for treatment; Europeans also underwent a similar fate. Unless the medical officers could cure insanity among Europeans, it was difficult for them to establish their credentials and control insanity amongst the 'natives'.

By 1861, the central building of the European Lunatic Asylum was partially repaired, and the wall around women's dormitories was thrown back. This increased the space of the courtyard. The Board anticipated that this would add to the ease and convenience of the female patients. But by 1892, as more female inmates were admitted, an upper storey of the building was added to avoid overcrowding. The medical officers of Bengal tried to offer the best accommodation for Europeans in Bengal. The purpose was to put the institution on a firm footing so that it could 'very well bear a comparison with one on a similar scale in Europe'.[94] Therefore, in this context, it is necessary to recognize the condition of the 'native' asylums and the situation of the inmates confined within them. Likewise, it is necessary to know the condition of patients in the 'native' asylums of Bengal, the rules and regulations implemented, and their mode of functioning. Some of the 'native' asylums discussed along the following lines include Russapaglah (Dullunda), Patna Lunatic Asylum, Dacca and Moorshedabad, Berhampore and Hazareebagh asylums, Moydapore Lunatic Asylum, and a proposed plan for a central lunatic asylum.

[93] Medical Board Proceedings, Number 53, Letter from Mrs Sims to K. Mackinon, 12 February 1853.

[94] Public Works Department, Number 19, 16 September 1853, Letter sent to Lord Dalhousie, Governor of Bengal from J. Thomson, Physician General and Charles Renny, Inspector General, Medical Board Office, dated 30 July 1853, NAI.

RUSSAPAGLAH (DULLUNDA) ASYLUM

Russapaglah, later known as Dullunda Asylum, was the oldest 'native' asylum of Bengal. A plan was sanctioned in 1804 to construct an asylum for 'natives' next to the Russa jail, in the 24 Parganas of Lower Bengal, for criminals and as well as those found 'freely wandering' on the streets. It was located on Russa Road in the southern suburbs of Calcutta, next to a jail. The hospital was built to house approximately fifty or sixty 'native' patients.[95] It was shifted to a new location closer to the river by 1847, and came to be known as Dullunda Asylum because of its new location in the 'fields of Dullunda' near Fort William.

This 'native' Insane Hospital was periodically visited by inspectors who were also members of the Medical Board. They were in charge of reporting on the overall functioning of the hospital. In most of the cases, while narrating the condition of the asylums of Bengal, the members of the Medical Board often showed their satisfaction over their own performances. For instance, I. Fleming, a member of the Medical Board, visited the hospital in 1811 and wrote to the Governor-General-in-Council:

> I found the business of the hospital properly conducted, every attention being paid to the patients in respect to their medical treatment diet, clothing and other circumstances conducive to their welfare and comfort as far as the nature of their respective cases will admit.[96]

At the time when the Russapaglah Asylum was newly built and the officers were constantly struggling to manage it, this statement was an exaggeration. Although the members of the Medical Board tried their utmost to manage the asylums there were severe lacunae in their modes of control and management, which they also tried to address. To begin with, they could never decide on a fixed place for the functioning of any of the asylums. Either the buildings constantly changed location or there was a constant need for extensions to the existing buildings. By 1813, it was realized that the space provided for the Insane Hospital

---

[95] Judicial Department, Criminal Branch Proceedings, Numbers 17–20, 1804, Letter sent by George Dowdeswell, Secretary to the Government of Bengal, Calcutta, Police Office, dated 5 August 1804, WBSA.

[96] Medical Board Proceedings, January 1811, Letter sent to Mr Tucker, Secretary to Government, Public Department by I. Fleming, First Member, Medical Board, dated 1 January 1811, NAI.

at Calcutta was insufficient. Therefore, the Public Department chose a site near Fort William for the construction of a new building, which included part of the old jail of Calcutta and part of the factory of Fort William for the 'reception and detention' of those persons whom the Supreme Court of Judicature at Fort William in Bengal would detain on account of their 'mental derangement'.[97] This illustrated that while the asylum makers thought of selecting a new site for the construction of asylums, they did not necessarily think of an unused or unsullied ground for the purpose. Often, abandoned buildings or parts of old buildings were transformed into asylums. For instance, in this case, parts of the jail and a factory were taken up for the construction of the asylum. The choice of location overlapping between a jail and a factory also had a connection with the definitions of insanity in the early nineteenth century, which considered vagabonds, destitutes, vagrants, and similar categories of socially dangerous people as insane. They were pulled out of the civilized population and admitted into asylums by the police on the recommendation of the Magistrate of the locality. The asylum was then considered more as a shelter, a place to hide the shame and disgrace of the society, than as a place for the treatment of mental illness. During the early nineteenth century, the asylum was mainly constituted of this heterogeneous crowd that intimidated the government because they did not fit into their definitions of 'normalcy'. Therefore, the location of an asylum next to a jail or the conversion of a jail into an asylum indicated overlapping of space; a space where both were confined for disciplining and treatment. Leonard Smith, while describing the public asylums of England in the early nineteenth century, had pointed out that 'custodial elements', which were central to the ideology of public asylums and 'curative aspirations' along with 'adoption of some principles of hospital architecture' were reflected in the construction of asylums during the time.[98]

[97] Medical Board Proceedings, February 1813, Letter sent to Charles Milner Ricketts, Secretary to Government Public Department by Edward Strettnell, Advocate General, dated 7 February 1813, NAI.

[98] Leonard Smith, 'The Architecture of Confinement: Urban Asylums in England, 1750–1820', in *Madness, Architecture and the Built Environment: Psychiatric Spaces in Historical Context*, edited by Leslie Topp, James E. Moran, and Jonathan Andrews (New York: Routledge, 2007), 43.

By 1815, the Insane Hospital of Calcutta was reallocated to a new building situated to the west of the old building.[99] In this new building, male and female patients were segregated, which, according to the Superintendent of the asylum, 'effected a change favourable on the minds of the patients of both sexes' as well as helped the medical officers to maintain the 'greatest decorum [in] the hospital'.[100] This segregation not only hinted that such divisions were maintained to guard issues of morality, but also gave birth to the beginning of the understanding of female insanity as separate from male. Hence, the difference in treatment also followed accordingly.

According to the medical practitioners, lack of space led to overcrowding, which, in turn, increased illness and delayed recovery. The number of inmates in all the 'native' asylums in the Lower Provinces of Bengal in most cases outnumbered the total cubic space designed for them. Shortly, the new building was found inappropriate because of the increasing death rate of patients, which in turn was related to the worsening condition of the hospital and the overcrowded situation within it. The increased mortality rate due to overcrowding was a common explanation put forth by almost all the superintendents of asylums throughout the nineteenth century. Mr Gillman, the Second Member of the Medical Board, visited the asylum in 1818 and reported,

> The site of it is very bad surrounded by jungle, swamps, *jeels*, pools from earth has been excavated for making bricks etc, etc. In short I believe, a worse situation could not be found. The buildings are low and damp and not half large enough for the number of patients, to which must be attributed the numerous deaths that occur there.[101]

Gillman, on his second visit to the Insane Hospital of Calcutta in June 1820, under the direction of the regulations for control and

[99] Judicial Proceedings, Criminal Branch, February 1815, Letter from John Eliot, Magistrate to W. B. Bayley, Acting Secretary to Government in the Judicial Department, dated 27 February 1815, WBSA.

[100] Judicial Proceedings, Criminal Branch, February 1815, Letter from H. Young, Surgeon to the Insane Hospital to John Eliot, Magistrate of the Suburbs of Calcutta, dated 11 July 1815, WBSA.

[101] Judicial Department, Criminal Branch Proceedings, Number 3, 1818, Letter sent by W. B. Bayley, Acting Chief Secretary to the Government of Bengal to the Secretary to the Medical Board, dated 17 March 1818, WBSA.

management of the asylum, provided a 'satisfactory report' as regards food, clothing, cleanliness, and treatment of the insane. His 'sentiments' on the 'damp, sultry and gloomy lower grounds' of the building closely surrounded by offices, walls, and trees was also taken into consideration by the Acting Chief Magistrate, H. Shakespear.[102] The Magistrate was not only in charge of sending a mentally ill person to an asylum, but also of inspecting asylums at regular intervals. However, his frequent absences from duty due to circumstances of an 'urgent and private nature' often caused difficulties in proper functioning of asylums.

A further addition was made to the building of the Insane Hospital of Calcutta by early 1821. An enclosed veranda of two floors with a staircase and walls with distinct boundaries between the two buildings was built. Cross walls were constructed within the compound to separate European patients from 'native' ones.[103] Although a separate asylum for European patients was built for their temporary stay by 1817, provisions were always maintained in the native asylums for the Europeans, Eurasians, and Anglo Indians. The option was kept open because European patients sent from the districts often temporarily lived in native asylums before they were shifted to the asylum specifically built for them. Second, Eurasian and Anglo-Indian patients who were also treated at the European hospital were often sent back to native asylums, when officers realized that they could not be sent back to England as they had no acquaintances there to take care of them. Hence, a part of the building was made especially for the Europeans with a dividing wall separating them from 'natives'. The number of European female inmates was always less than the number of 'native' insane women admitted in the Insane Hospital, although the former had the privilege of staying in a separate building specifically built for them. In contrast, 'native' women, although confined to separate wings, did not have the advantage of a separate building exclusively meant for their treatment in as early as 1820s. The number of 'native' insane women in each cell often outnumbered its capacity. The situation improved by

[102] Medical Board Proceedings, 9 August 1820, Letter sent to C. Lushington, Secretary to Government in General Department by J. Gillman, Second Member of Medical Board, Calcutta, dated 1 July 1820, NAI.

[103] Medical Board Proceedings, February 1821, Letter sent to three members of the Medical Board, W. Ogilvy, I. Gillman, and I. Meik by J. Sawers, Superintendent of the Insane Hospital, dated February 1821, NAI.

the mid-nineteenth century, when a separate wing for 'native' women was constructed in the Patna Lunatic Asylum.

In 1838, the Surgeon of the 24 Parganas expressed his apprehension about the poor condition of the Insane Hospital at Calcutta in a letter to the Magistrate. The Hospital, according to him, had not undergone any renovation work in the previous two decades. His description of the state of affairs not only expressed his concern for the condition of the hospital, but also showed the incapability of the decision makers to devise an ideal situation of an asylum and its inmates, which they constantly tried to derive from their understanding of the European asylums. The ceiling of the asylum leaked considerably. The ground floor, which had never been properly repaired since the erection of the building, was in a bad state. Therefore, to avoid sleeping on the damp floor, *machan*s made of bamboo were constructed by the inmates, which they used to sleep on at night. He further reported the status of doors and verandas, which according to him not only required mending but also needed new bolts and locks. The beams required paint and the drains required renovation. To improve the situation, in July he recommended two more significant changes within the asylum. First, the construction of 'air holes above the ceiling', and second, a 'screen' in the central ward, under the four windows facing the women's apartments, so as to prevent the female patients looking into the men's compound from their machans.[104] Suggestions to make open holes in the ceiling for proper air circulation not only revealed the congested situation within the cells, but also pointed to severe lacunae in the imagination of the medical officers. Making holes in the ceilings and allowing rainwater to seep through when it rained made inmates more susceptible to illnesses. The same logic would also follow during winter when cold air entering through these holes made them fall sick. This also illustrated that without having a proper understanding of the situation and the available infrastructure, they often took decisions for the care of the patients, that proved to be fatal.

When the Surgeon, who was thoughtful about the refurbishment of wards and verandas, urgently requested the Civil Architect to take necessary measures, the Civil Architect on the contrary considered certain

---

[104] Medical Board Proceedings, 18 February 1839, Letter sent to J. H. Patton, Magistrate, 24 Parganas by F. P. Strong, Surgeon 24 Parganas, dated 12 July 1838, NAI.

other modifications as more important. These included filed choppers, sky lights, venations, iron gratings, and the privies other than *pukka* flooring of the several wards and verandas.[105] Differences of opinion between a Civil Architect and a medical person not only made the inmates a pawn in the game but the contradiction also showed that it was not only the opinion of the medical professionals but also that of a Civil Architect that contributed towards the understanding of the condition of the asylums and its patients. After proposals for several new additions to the building by the Superintendent, the renovation work was finally limited to only 'painting and plastering' of the asylum and no attention was paid to the floors and verandas,[106] not to mention the drains. Thus, despite the concern conveyed by the Surgeon, the reconstruction of the asylum was limited to its outer decoration, which was an illusory attempt to prove that the institution was in a 'good' condition.

Yet by 1839, renovation work remained incomplete because the Surgeon did not sign the total estimate for repairs sent to Captain Fitzgeralds, the Civil Architect at Fort William. The Civil Architect differed in his opinion from the Surgeon, and therefore, only made general repairs of the wards and verandas and cemented the compound. Once the work got over, it was realized that verandas and wards had holes in them. This created an unhealthy atmosphere because not only did the water that was used to clean the floors accumulate in it, but the holes were also covered by the waste thrown out by patients especially at night, all of which together got absorbed in the holes and gave off bad odour. Therefore, the Surgeon requested the Board not to use chunar stone, which had been in use since 1819, any further. Chunar stone caused dampness because of its porosity.[107] The difference in opinion proved

[105] Medical Board Proceedings 18 February 1839, Letter sent to F. Strong, Surgeon, 24 Parganas by Captain Fitzgerald, Civil Architect, Fort William, dated 20 April 1838, NAI.

[106] Medical Board Proceedings, 18 February 1839, Letter sent to John Master, Judge and Magistrate, 24 Parganas by F. P. Strong, Surgeon 24 Parganas, dated 12 July 1838, NAI.

[107] Medical Board Proceedings, 18 February 1839, Letter sent to Colin Campbell, Third Member of the Medical Board and Superintending Surgeon, Calcutta Division by F. P. Strong, Surgeon, 24 Parganas, dated 7 February 1839, NAI.

disadvantageous to patients who had to suffer because of it. Inmates therefore slept on the machan, which was a raised platform, until the repair work got over.[108] The Civil Architect was unaware of the right material for proper flooring. Also, there were probably not enough funds available for proper construction.

By 1843 the Board decided to construct a new building with a capacity of thirty patients in addition to the number of patients already in confinement at Russapaglah. It further recommended the most complete separation of the sexes inside the asylum, not only by a railing or wall, but, if possible, by locating them on separate sides of the building. The Board objected to the site of the existing hospital on Russa Road, because of three reasons. First, distance from the centre of the town; second, the site was on a low ground; third, because of the small area, the rooms were too confined.[109] According to J. P. Strong, the increase in the number of inmates in the asylum sent by the Magistrate made it impossible to keep the wards and verandas clean, which prevented the recovery of patients, many of whom, he believed, would have otherwise recovered and returned to their families.[110] He further stated that the number of deaths in the Insane Hospitals of France, England, and Europe was higher than in India. This, according to him, should have been the opposite because the former countries had the 'advantages of a superior climate'.[111] This showed that by the 1840s, the medical officers did not only conclude that mortality was higher among Europeans and 'natives' in India due to the climatic conditions, but, the 'negative character of the Asiatics' who, due to their ignorance, were only admitted to asylums during the 'last stages of mental imbecility and

[108] Medical Board Proceedings, Number 18A, 3 April 1843, Letter sent to John Marshall, Inspector General of Hospital Presidency by J. P. Strong, Surgeon, 24 Parganas, dated 31 March 1843, NAI.

[109] Medical Board Proceedings, Number 4, 2 February 1843, Letter sent to the Deputy Governor of Bengal Medical Board by C. Campbell and J. Marshall, Members of the Medical Board, dated 31 January 1843, NAI.

[110] Medical Board Proceedings Number 18A, Letter from J. P. Strong to John Marshall, 31 March 1843.

[111] Medical Board Proceedings Number 18A, Letter from J. P. Strong to John Marshall, 31 March 1843.

corporal suffering combined',[112] thus causing mortality in the asylums of India.

Finally in 1847, the Insane Hospital was removed and relocated to a separate building, in the near vicinity of the old Insane Hospital, in Dullunda, to the south of Fort William, between Alipore and Bhawanipore, and in the immediate vicinity of the latter suburbs. The proposal for building a new Asylum in 1843 finally took shape in 1847. The new building was spacious than the previous one. Hence, more patients were accommodated in it than before.[113] According to the Board, although the building was raised much before that time, two things hindered the process of displacement. First, there was a delay in erecting the external compound wall resulting in it being unoccupied during the rains; second, the new building was built on lower ground, which produced dampness, because unlike other wards and verandas, the floors of the new building were not covered with asphalt. Therefore, the moist surroundings of the asylum provided space for the growth of weeds, thus damaging the construction.[114] This illustrated that while they had the knowledge, they failed to implement it into practice due to lack of infrastructure. To control the situation, the Surgeon of the 24 Parganas recommended to the Chief Engineer that the ground level of the hospital, independent of the foundation, be elevated by at least 5 to 6 feet.[115] Although the orders were very prompt, their implementation always took a longer period and in many instances remained unexecuted.

The site of Dullunda Asylum was considered suitable by the Board because it was airy as well as exposed to the north of the plain surrounding Fort William, while the south front was kept open by the grounds of the asylum. The building for male patients was made of four wings. It faced

[112] Medical Board Proceedings Number 18A, Letter from J. P. Strong to John Marshall, 31 March 1843.

[113] 'Annual Report on the Lunatic Asylums for the European and Native Insane Patients at Bhawanipore and Dullunda for 1856 and 1857,' in *Selections from the Records of the Government of Bengal*, Number XXVIII (Calcutta: John Gray, 1858), NAI.

[114] 'Report on Insane Hospital at Calcutta, by the Surgeon of the Twenty Four Parganas' sent to the Inspector General of Hospitals, 1847, National Library, Kolkata [henceforth NL].

[115] 'Report on Insane Hospital at Calcutta,' 1847.

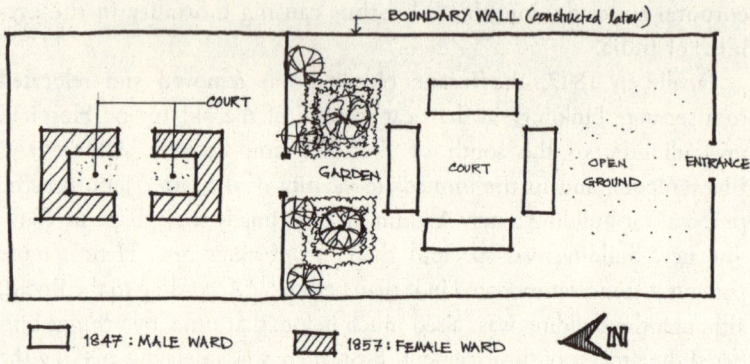

Figure 1.1   Dullunda Asylum
Source: Author.

a large square court, and stood between a garden and the open grounds
to the south. A separate building for female inmates was constructed and
opened almost ten years later in April 1857 (see Figure 1.1). A boundary
wall, with an entrance from the garden, separated the building from
the adjoining one for males. This house for female patients was erected
between two airy courts and faced both north and south directions.
Rooms were lofty and the foundation was more elevated than the rest
of the asylum. The wards and verandas formed three sides of a square,
which opened to the southern courtyard. According to the superintendent, such a design was made in order to secure a thorough air flow in
between the corridors. The eight dormitories, of which one was used
as a hospital, were built along the design similar to that of the division
for males. A kitchen was erected at one end of the courtyard. Both the
courtyard and the veranda provided grounds for labour, occupation,
and exercise. Refractory wards were not constructed in the new asylum.
During paroxysms of violence, female inmates were not secluded, but
were confined to one of the dormitories.[116]

Although additions to the buildings commenced in the early
part of 1869, the work was stopped abruptly due to fiscal restraints.
Therefore, by 1870, the northern extensions of the building were

[116] *Annual Report on the Lunatic Asylums for the European and Native Insane
Patients at Bhawanipore and Dullunda for 1856 and 1857.*

carried up to the floor level only. Several feet of walls were added to the building where the female wards were situated. This resulted in great inconvenience for the officers. According to A. Payne, as the building was close to the level of the boundary wall, female inmates often used it as a means of escape. Although this was reported to the public works department and an urgent request submitted for the completion of that portion of the building, 'no further progress' was made.[117] Delay in prompt action during such an emergency pointed to the incapability of the administrators, while also confirming their lackadaisical attitude towards the maintenance of the inmates.

Throughout the nineteenth century, asylum buildings were continually built and rebuilt. At times, the site of the asylum was changed, and at other times, extensions were made to the existing buildings. In 1870, the Superintendent of Dullunda Asylum reported that the female wards were expanded and new cooking and eating sheds were also made. Perforated zinc was applied to protect the interior of the cook room as well as the 'eating sheds' to avoid flies and other 'vermin'.[118] Another building was completed by 1871 within the same compound. Even an extension of the existing building did not resolve the problem of space. This was reflected in the words of the Superintendent of the asylum, A. Payne:

> The massing together of lunatics certainly imports difficulties into the question of their proper control and treatment, especially when space is limited, or has only been intended, or is adapted, for comparatively small numbers.[119]

[117] 'Report on Dullunda Asylum for the Year 1869,' by Surgeon Major Arthur Payne, Superintendent of Asylums at the Presidency sent to Deputy Inspector General of Hospitals, Presidency Circle, Fort William, Dullunda, January 1870, in *Annual Report on the Insane Asylums in Bengal, 1869* by J. Murray, Inspector General of Hospitals, Indian Medical Department (Calcutta: Bengal Secretariat Office, 1870), NAI.

[118] *General Report Number 3 on the Lunatic Asylums, Vaccinations and Dispensaries in the Bengal Presidency for the Year 1870,* compiled by Assistant Surgeon K. McLeod, A. M., M. D., Officiating Secretary to the Inspector General of Hospitals, Indian Medical Department (Calcutta: Bengal Secretariat Press, 1872), NAI.

[119] Letter Number 346 from J. Campbell Brown, Inspector General of Hospitals, Indian Medical Department to the Officiating Secretary to the Government of Bengal, Fort William, dated 27 June 1872, *Annual Report on the Insane Asylums in Bengal for the Year 1871.*

Regardless of the structure of the new building, overcrowding in the asylums continued. Surgeon R. Bird, in the annual report, stated that there were

> fifty superficial feet for each patient—and lunatics should not have less—the asylum can only contain 293 lunatics, while the daily average in confinement exceeded this number by 61.[120]

Lack of space within an asylum caused more difficulty for female inmates than men. First, their sleeping rooms were more crowded than that of men; second, their courtyards, in proportion to their number, were smaller and more confined; third, the workshed in the women's courtyard was not only small but also did not have a shade to protect them from the sun. Moreover, the courtyard was insufficiently ventilated. The asylum officials endeavoured to create a better situation for the inmates, but failed to keep up with the constant provisions that had to be made.

THE PATNA LUNATIC ASYLUM

An Insane Hospital for soldiers was established at Monghyr in Bihar in the late eighteenth century. During that time there was an influx of troops into the hospital who were both physically and mentally ill. The hospital failed to cope with this entry because of the dearth of 'expert' medical officers as well as lack of medical aid to Monghyr. Thus, on 8 September 1795, the Lieutenant Colonel commanding at Monghyr proposed to the Adjutant General the establishment of an Insane Hospital in Patna along with a full-time Surgeon in order to reduce the burden on the former hospital.[121] By 1820, the Insane Hospital at Patna shifted to a new building because the old building failed to accommodate the number of patients admitted to it. Women's apartments were separated from men's by a partition wall about 8-feet high. The new building was built without a compound wall surrounding it. A concrete drain was also absent. The Superintending Surgeon believed that a compound wall and a concrete drain would make the asylum

[120] Remarks on Several Asylums of Bengal, *Annual Report on the Insane Asylums in Bengal for the Year 1872.*

[121] Medical Board Proceedings, 20 January 1796, Letter sent to Lieutenant Colonel Murray, Adjutant General by Lieutenant Colonel E. Ellerker commanding at Monghyr, NAI.

complete for the 'purposes of which it was intruded by Government'.[122] In 1823, a proposal was submitted for the construction of a new hospital for women with ventilators on the roof instead of large holes in the ceilings that had been previously constructed for ventilation. A proposal was also made to construct a boundary wall around the already existing hospital for male patients in the city of Patna. In order to accommodate 'servants', who usually occupied the entrance of the veranda, the Board proposed that a small building be constructed next to the main asylum building to be used as servants' quarters.[123]

The majority of insane were described by the medical officers on admission as extremely weak and emaciated, and also as having suffered from 'neglect and harsh treatment'. Their condition, according to J. Sutherland, became different after a few weeks' residence in the asylum: many became 'stout and healthy' under careful treatment. Daily oil massage for patients who appeared to be in a perfectly hopeless state on admission was considered beneficial. This was particularly so in the case of those patients whose skin became rough and dry. Under such circumstances, 'oil friction' was known to improve general health.[124]

According to J. Forsyth, the site of the Patna Lunatic Asylum was ill chosen (see Figures 1.2 and 1.3). Hence, the asylum inmates suffered during floods and the building was damaged. He was anxious about the recurrence of such events.[125] The inmates had already been suffering from cholera before the flood, and the consequences that followed were even worse. The water rose to such a level that it flooded the cells and submerged the water tank within the courtyard. As the surrounding

[122] Medical Board Proceedings, July 1820, Letter sent to J. Jameson by Robert Lowe, Superintending Surgeon, dated 5 July 1820, NAI.

[123] Medical Board Proceedings, 2 July 1823, Letter sent to W. B. Bayley, Chief Secretary to Government by George Proctor, Secretary Medical Board, dated 30 June 1823, NAI.

[124] Bengal Proceedings, Medical Department, Number 38, 27 February 1861, in *Report on Patna Lunatic Asylum for the Year 1860* by J. Sutherland, Civil Surgeon, APAC, BL.

[125] General Proceedings, Medical Department, February 1862, in *Annual Report of the Insane Hospital at Patna for the Year 1861* sent to E. H. Lushington, Secretary to the Government of Bengal from J. Forsyth, Principal Inspector General, Medical Department, WBSA.

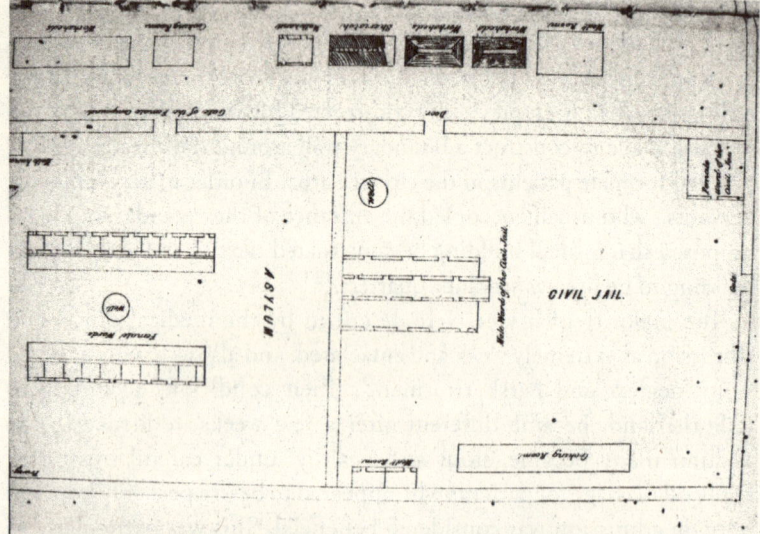

Figure 1.2 Diagram of Patna Lunatic Asylum Showing the 'Female Ward'
Source: Author.

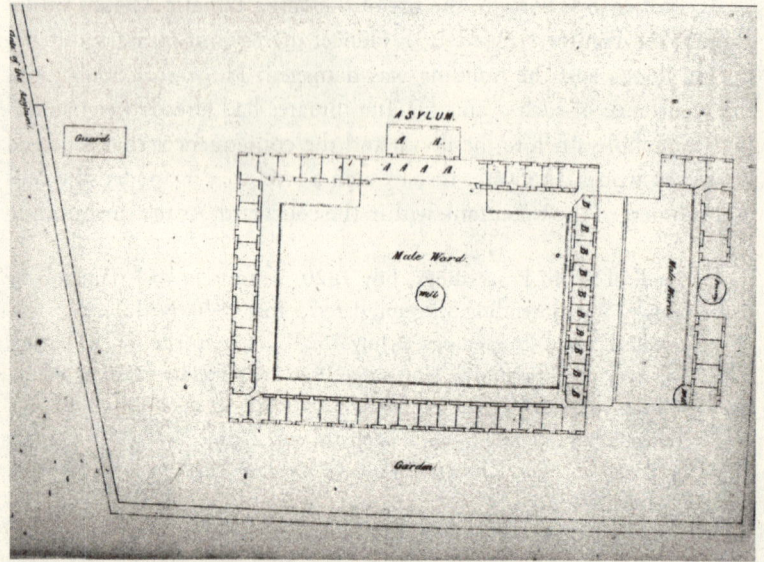

Figure 1.3 Diagram of Patna Lunatic Asylum Showing the 'Male Ward'
Source: Author.

grounds became marshy, the floors of the cells remained damp and wet for several months. In order to resolve the problem, asylums had the provision of 'stoves' for drying cells and wards. Nevertheless, reports never stated the safety measures adopted for its functioning in the presence of asylum inmates. Equipment of this sort could expose mentally challenged people to various risk factors. It is difficult to assume how the asylum administrators visualized its usage and thereby implemented necessary safety measures.

Sanitation and hygiene conditions often worsened during the rainy season when water stagnated outside the asylum gate and rose above the level of the drain. Drainage plans and construction were supervised by the Public Works Department. Often, lack of asylum funds for the maintenance of the asylum led to ill or unfinished constructions, which affected the inhabitants of the asylums. Hence severe bowel complaints prevailed up to the middle of December. Most of the patients who were victims of the disease were feeble 'imbeciles' with chronic organic diseases.[126] Under these circumstances the Inspector General of Hospitals was apprehensive that the situation would worsen in case there was another flood unless necessary steps were taken. Therefore, he requested the government to look into the matter. Although the government had initially approved the construction of another asylum on a 'better site' with an improved plan—as the existing building demanded a lot of renovation work and the site was considered unfit for the well-being of its inmates[127]—it refused after inspection stating that the building was not a 'bad one' and that the lack of public service in other sectors made it impossible to construct another new building.[128] The Inspector General of Hospitals, who

[126] Bengal Proceedings, Medical Department, Number 43, 27 February 1862, Letter sent to E. H. Lushington, Secretary to the Government of Bengal from J. Forsyth, Principal Inspector General, Medical Department, dated 18 February 1862, APAC, BL.

[127] Bengal Proceedings, Medical Department, Number 43, Letter from J. Forsyth to E. H. Lushington, 18 February 1862.

[128] Bengal Proceedings, Medical Department, Number 46, 27 February 1862, Letter sent to the Principal Inspector General, Medical Department from H. Bell, Officiating Junior Secretary to the Government of Bengal, dated 27 February 1862, APAC, BL.

was also a medical professional, often failed to convince the adminis-
trator about the necessity for better arrangements for the well-being
of the patients.

Death rates at the asylum varied. In 1861, according to Dr Guise, the
superintendent of the Patna Lunatic Asylum, the decrease in mortality
rate was due to the improved sanitary condition.[129] In another instance,
in 1897, the reason for low mortality according to the Superintendent
was that greater care was taken of each individual case, 'both when well
and sick', and also because prophylactics were given twice a week to all
inmates of the asylum.[130] But in 1900, when there was an increase in the
death rate at the Patna Asylum, it was attributed to the general ill health
of the town and district.[131]

DACCA AND MOORSHEDABAD LUNATIC ASYLUMS

In 1805, a proposal was submitted to the government for the construction of an asylum at Dacca (see Figure 1.4).[132] The plan envisaged cells
measuring 6 feet by 6 feet and a compound of 4 feet by 6 feet covered
with a thatched roof. The Surgeon of the 24 Parganas in a letter to
His Majesty's Justices of Peace for the town of Calcutta argued against
such a small place allotted for the asylum. Rather, he offered a design
that included seven cells spanning 12 feet by 8 feet each along with
a veranda and another set of fourteen cells of 10 feet by 7 feet. The
Surgeon also proposed to replace the combustible thatched roof with
a concrete structure. In order to make a future provision for an upper
storey building he suggested roof walls of 2-feet thickness. Otherwise,

[129] Bengal Proceedings, Medical Department, Number 5, 4 February 1862,
Letter sent to the Government of Bengal, to the Principal Inspector General,
Medical Department from H. Bell, Officiating Junior Secretary to the Govern-
ment of Bengal, dated 4 February 1862, APAC, BL.

[130] *Annual Report of the Lunatic Asylums of Bengal for the Year 1898* by
Colonel T. H. Hendeley.

[131] Home Department, Medical Branch, Number 52, September 1900,
'Annual Report on the Lunatic Asylums of India for 1899,' by E. N. Baker.

[132] Judicial Proceedings, Criminal Branch, May 1805, Letter from
F. Martyn and W. Blaquiere to G. Dawdeswell, Secretary to Government,
Calcutta Police Office, dated 26 April 1805, WBSA.

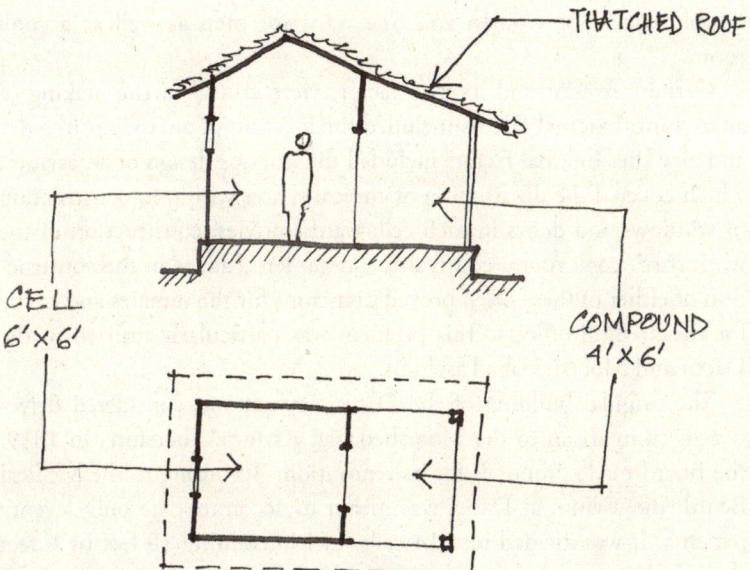

Figure 1.4 Diagram of Dacca Lunatic Asylum, 1805
Source: Author.

walls measuring 1.6-feet and the 16-inch thick partition walls between each cell were thought of as sufficient. Iron doors measuring about 6 feet by 3 feet were built for each cell instead of closed doors to keep the patients under absolute observation at any time of the day. Curtains were tied to the doors to combat cold during winter. The windows were 3 feet by 3 feet, and built at a height of 6 feet above the ground. Similar sized windows were also used in the cook room. The Surgeon pointed out the necessity of two separate compounds for male and female patients, but it was never executed as it was not drawn in the initial plan of the asylum.[133] In 1819, an extension of the asylum was taken into consideration, and a piece of land owned by the Nawab of Dacca was considered by the Board as the most convenient place for this purpose. The Nawab sanctioned the land. The Board proposed

[133] Judicial Proceedings, Criminal Branch, May 1805, Letter from C. Cornish, Surgeon, 24 Parganas to His Majesty's Justices of the Peace for the Town of Calcutta, dated 25 April 1805, WBSA.

double wards for women and one ward for men as well as a cook room.[134]

Certain exterior and interior factors were crucial in the making of an asylum. External factors included the location of an asylum in a dry and airy site. Internal factors included the interior design of an asylum, which covered the distribution of cubical spaces within it, construction of windows and doors in each cell, wards, privies, construction of the work shed, cook room, courtyard, and garden. Failure in the construction of either of these often proved disastrous for the inmates and tricky for the medical officers. This problem was particularly realized in the Dacca and Moorshedabad asylums.

The original building of the Dacca Asylum was considered defective in comparison to the Moorshedabad Asylum. Therefore, in 1819, the Board made proposals for its renovation. According to the Medical Board, the asylum at Dacca was meant to accommodate only seventy patients. It was divided into 14 cells, each measuring 10 feet by 6 feet each, and two wards—one measuring 58 feet by 16 feet for men, and a smaller one measuring 20 feet by 16 feet for women. Fourteen patients were accommodated in the cells and the remaining fifty-six were distributed in the two wards, which together measured only 78 feet by 16 feet. Therefore, it provided space for little more than 22 superficial square feet to each patient. The size of each cell was considered too small particularly in a place with a hot climate like India. Therefore, the superintendent recommended cells of a size not less than 10 feet by 8 feet. But other than the size of cells, its distribution was also an important factor. There were seven cells, 20 feet wide, on each side of a narrow court, placed immediately opposite each other (see Figure 1.5). The disadvantage caused due to the close arrangement of cells, as stated by the Surgeon, was that as a result of being so close, every word spoken on one side was heard and every action was seen by those on the opposite side. Therefore, whenever any patient became out of control and noisy, it irritated those on the opposite side and rendered them worse and equally noisy.

The windows of both Dacca and Moorshedabad Asylums were described as 'too small and too high'. The outer windows had only bars.

[134] Medical Board Proceedings, Number 31, 13 April 1819, Letter sent to James Jameson, Secretary to the Medical Board from T. Phipps, Superintendent of Building Works, NAI.

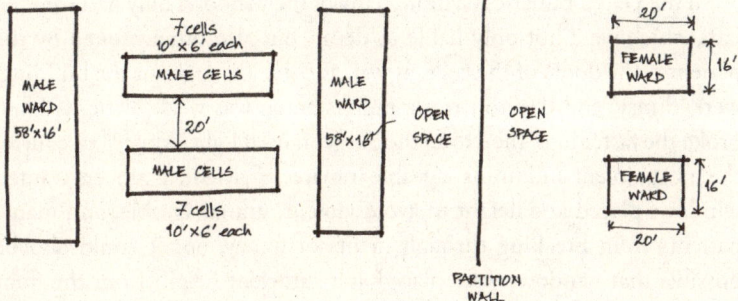

Figure 1.5 Diagram of Dacca Lunatic Asylum, as Proposed in 1819
Source: Author.

This was a 'bad plan' as the patients constantly tried to tear them from their hinges.[135] According to the Surgeon of the Moorshedabad Asylum, the windows ought to have been on the outside with shutters, so that they would fold back upon the wall and be shut from outside in order to prevent the patients from reaching them. These kinds of windows were suggested instead of *jhānp*s,[136] which were initially used but later found ineffective as they failed to protect inmates from the cold in winter or from rain during the rainy season. Therefore, changes in the weather affected the patients and they often complained of bowel problems during these seasons. To combat such difficulties, windows were replaced as per the Surgeon's proposal. Moreover, the Moorshedabad Insane Hospital had fixed venetian blinds besides the bars instead of windows. The Surgeon had also opposed the construction of small windows at a height from the floor, in both men's and women's wards. For reasons of safety and security, the medical officer of the hospital suggested the construction of a wall around the well, with a door to lock and a trough to supply water to the patients. This was to 'preclude the necessity of their having any direct communication with the wells'.[137]

[135] Home Department, Medical Board Proceedings, Number 39, 11 June 1821, Letter sent to James Jameson, Secretary to the Medical Board, Calcutta from Alexander Russell, Superintending Surgeon, Berhampore, dated 25 May 1821, NAI.

[136] 'Jhānp' is a hurdle of matting and bamboo, used as a shutter or door.

[137] Home Department, Medical Board Proceedings, Number 39, Letter from Alexander Russell to James Jameson, 25 May 1821.

In the Dacca Lunatic Asylum, many of the windows only had wooden bars which were not only liable to decay, but also often broken by the patients. The doors of the cells, as well as those throughout the building, were 'flimsy' and the iron work and fastening was weak. Patients often broke the fastening. Therefore, the Surgeon used light irons[138] to control the most violent and unmanageable inmates.[139] Medical officers wanted windows placed at a height to avoid violent, unmanageable, and manic patients from breaking through in fits of frenzy, but it could also be possible that windows were placed at a sufficient height from the floor so that 'lunatics' could not use them as escape routes.

In the Moorshedabad Lunatic Asylum there were only fourteen cells and one ward for men. Therefore, once the cells were occupied, patients were all clustered together in the remaining ward, which included the curable and incurable, the violent and calm, the filthy and clean, and the furious and the melancholy. This caused difficulty in treatment. Often single cells were combined and turned into one enlarged cell.[140] This not only hindered proper treatment of patients, but also blurred the dividing lines of classification of patients into separate categories. Convalescent wards were constructed for the treatment of violent inmates. The intention of the physicians was to prevent their relapses thereby ensuring permanent recovery. Due to lack of space, it was not possible to maintain one patient in one ward. Therefore, in the Moorshedabad Asylum, convalescent wards were of 'little or no use' as they failed to serve the purpose.[141] A crowded single ward was dangerous for the treatment of any chronic or contagious diseases amongst inmates. Since diarrhoea was very frequent inside the asylum, the provision of a separate cell for each patient was thought of as a better alternative by the Surgeon of the asylum.

The idea of separate cells was fully supported by the concurring testimonies of many eminent physicians of great experience in Europe

[138] 'Light iron' is a kind of shackling device, used to restrain violent patients.

[139] Medical Board Proceedings, May 1821, Letter sent to James Jameson, Secretary Medical Board by Alexander Russell, Superintending Surgeon Berhampore, dated 25 May 1821, NAI.

[140] Medical Board Proceedings, Letter from Alexander Russell to James Jameson, 25 May 1821.

[141] Medical Board Proceedings, Letter from Alexander Russell to James Jameson, 25 May 1821.

and thoroughly confirmed by the personal observations of the Board in the Bareilly and Russapaglah hospitals, which were considered the two largest establishments of this description in the nineteenth century. The ideal method of treatment lay not only in the harsh and indiscriminate confinement of patients or in their 'jumbling' together but in a balance between the two extremes.[142]

At Dacca, two wards for women were built at a distance from each other. Each of these rooms measured 20 feet by 16 feet. A partition wall separated the women's division from that of the men's. But no separate cells or apartments were constructed either in women's or men's divisions. An open space was allocated for the inmates' exercise and recreation (see Figure 1.6). In the Moorshedabad Asylum, a partition wall separated the women's division from the men's but it was constructed so close to the cell that it impeded free circulation of air.

For 'punishing' patients, the superintendent demanded the construction of five or six cells separated from the main building but within the compound. Although this was meant to control violent and noisy patients, it was also designed to house those inmates who

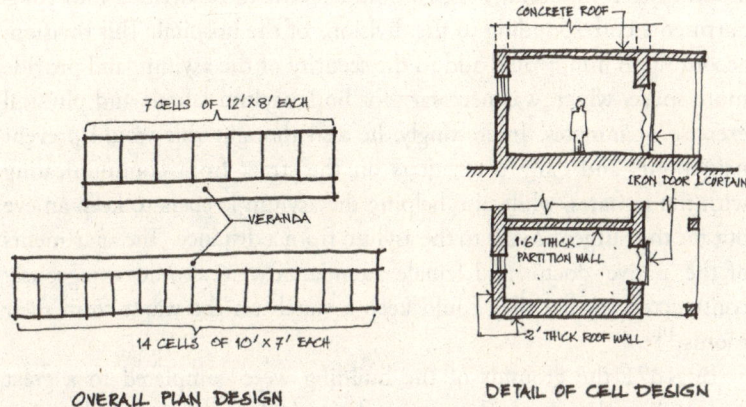

Figure 1.6 Dacca Asylum: Proposal by Surgeon of the 24 Parganas
Source: Author.

[142] Medical Board Proceedings, June 1821, Letter sent to Bayley, Chief Secretary to Government by J. Jameson, Secretary Medical Board, dated 12 June 1821, NAI.

committed any 'fault', hence the 'punishment'. The construction of the new building was proposed with a veranda built on both sides of the cells. The system of 'checks and control' was introduced at both Moorshedabad and Dacca Asylums to provide comfort to the patients and secure due attention to their wants. The system also helped to keep check on the medical establishment in the asylum and their control on the patients.[143]

By 1842, the Insane Hospital at Moorshedabad had three wards. The main ward with fifty-six cells and a separate room capable of accommodating twelve patients were constructed for male patients, and a smaller ward to the north built for the convalescent, noisy, and unruly patients who were found guilty of any criminal offence and also for those criminal inmates who were detained for further trial while under the treatment of mental illness.

The female ward with only ten cells was constructed at the southern end. Although the Surgeon approved of the hospital being situated in a 'healthy' surrounding, he found the construction defective. Therefore, certain modifications were proposed. First, construction of a dividing wall through the centre of the main ward; second, a wall to be built around the compound, which would allow it to be divided into compartments corresponding to the divisions of the hospital. This division, according to him, would add to the security of the asylum, and provide more space, which was necessary for both asylum labour and physical exercise of inmates. Interestingly, he also thought this would prevent neighbours and daily commuters on the street from communicating with the inmates, while also helping the asylum keepers to keep an eye out for the Surgeon's visit to the asylum from a distance. The apartments of the 'native' doctor and female attendants were also advantageously constructed so that they could keep a watch on the wards from their rooms.[144]

By 1871 the grounds of the building were completed to a great extent. A garden was laid out with flower beds and for the cultivation

[143] Medical Board Proceedings, Letter from Alexander Russell to James Jameson, 25 May 1821.

[144] Medical Board Proceedings, May 1842, Letter sent to W. Findon, Superintending Surgeon Presidency Division by A. Kean, Secretary to the Government of India, dated 15 September 1841, NAI.

of vegetables, to give a 'cheerful' appearance to the institution, thereby removing all ideas of 'gloom and restraint'.[145] The wards were well-ventilated, with provisions for sufficient light and air to flow in. The female ward consisted of verandas, divided into compartments for two patients each, and was separated from the rest of the asylum by a partition wall. A masonry drain was made through the premises, and the ground was improved by filling up holes, levelling, and planting trees and shrubs.[146]

In 1875, the Deputy Surgeon General of the Dacca circle, Dr J. C. Bow, asserted that high mortality among female inmates was caused by the 'excessive and draughty ventilation'. During the same year, a large number of patients were diagnosed with bowel irregularities, which the superintendent assumed was due to the poor quality of food and water supply, insufficient amount of clothing provided, and dampness in the sleeping wards.[147] Hence, a new ward to accommodate forty patients was constructed in the following year. It was a pukka building, which rose on arches and had a south veranda extending along its entire length. The building was divided into twelve cells, four to accommodate sixteen patients and eight to accommodate twenty-four patients; each cell was furnished with two opposite doors. It was situated in the garden to the west of the other buildings, and water well previously in use was removed from the other buildings. In 1876, the superintendent mentioned that although there was deficiency in accommodation, it did not affect the standard of health of the inmates. The greatest average number of mentally ill patients were admitted in January, and the least in October. Thus, the change in weather conditions and not the lack of space were seen as a significant factor by the asylum officers for this variation in admission.

[145] Wise, 'Report on the Dacca Lunatic Asylum,' *Annual Report on the Lunatic Asylums of Bengal for the Year 1871*.

[146] Wise, 'Report on the Dacca Lunatic Asylum,' *Annual Report on the Lunatic Asylums of Bengal for the Year 1871*.

[147] Surgeon D. B. Smith, 'Report on the Dacca Lunatic Asylum for the Year 1876,' *Annual Report on the Insane Asylums of Bengal for the Year 1876*, by J. Fullarton Beatson, Surgeon General, Indian Medical Department to Secretary to the Government of Bengal Judicial Department, Fort William, 16 July 1877 (Calcutta: Bengal Secretariat Press, 1877), NAI.

BERHAMPORE AND HAZAREEBAGH LUNATIC ASYLUMS

Overlapping of spaces often occurred during the construction of asylums. Often an old jail or an abandoned military barrack was converted into an asylum, as it was in the case of the Berhampore Asylum when it was established in 1876. The asylum at Berhampore had a capacity of housing 147 male and 55 female patients, while the largest numbers in confinement on any one night at the asylum consisted of 163 men and 59 women. The asylum was always found to be overcrowded, owing to the peculiar construction of the barracks, which were originally built for European soldiers. It was also because of the lack of a sufficient number of solitary cells for the separate confinement of noisy and dangerous inmates. Thus, whenever physicians thought it necessary to put a patient in solitary confinement, one of the smaller wards was emptied, and its inmates, numbering eight or ten, were distributed among the other wards, which already received as many occupants as they could accommodate. This undesirable condition caused inconveniences. According to the Inspector General of Hospitals, it had put the inmates at serious risk of injury to their health. Therefore, he requested the government to extend the building, so as to provide a suitable site for solitary cells at some distance from the main buildings.[148]

In the twenty-first century, this asylum is known as Beharampur Mental Hospital.[149] It is still maintained by the government. The old building which was previously used as a prison to accommodate both inmates of the jail and the asylum is at present abandoned. Separate buildings are constructed for men and women. While in the women's building, women of different age groups and categories of illnesses are roomed together, in the men's quarters the situation is different. In the latter three-storied building, men are classified in

[148] Home, Medical, Number 135, July 1890, Letter sent to the Chief Secretary to the Government of Bengal from A. Hilson, Inspector General of Civil Hospitals, Bengal, dated 8 April 1890, NAI.

[149] I visited the Beharampur Mental Hospital in December, 2012 and its description in the following lines is how I found it at present. It shows how far and if at all the condition of the mentally ill, their treatment, or for that matter even the construction of the building has changed since the nineteenth century.

each of the floors not on the basis of class or caste differences but on the basis of their age group. 'Solitary confinement', a term often used in the medical documents on asylums of the nineteenth century, is replaced by the term 'observatory ward' in the twenty-first century. During the nineteenth century, these special confinement areas were characterized as small dark rooms with no ventilation and a toilet in one corner. In the present day, these rooms are more airy with one big window, a ceiling fan (although covered with iron fencing), and a toilet-cum-bathroom attached to the ward. Ceiling fans in all the rooms of both male and female wards are covered with iron fencing in order to avoid any kind of self-damage by the patients. This hospital does not engage its patients in any labour activity. The only source of entertainment is television, provided in each of the dormitory rooms. While the women's building has only one dining hall as all of them are kept on one single floor only, the men's building has separate dining halls on each floor. There are female nurses in both the buildings. A senior female nurse from the men's building allowed me to visit the third floor of the building which accommodated men of age forty-five and above. She was apprehensive of my visit on other floors which housed younger mentally unfit men. Overall, she commented that women patients are easier to handle than male patients of any age. The superintendent of the asylum lamented that irrespective of the fact that so many of them got cured, they still continued to stay 'inside' as they had no place to return to. I personally interacted with many of the patients in the women's ward. They not only responded but very clearly recalled their family and place of residence, about their children back home, their relatives, and friends. They also told me that they know they have no place to return to and there is nobody waiting for them back at home because they were diagnosed as mentally ill. They are also aware of the fact that nurses only 'console' them as well as others who are yet to be cured that someday they would be released from their confinement and would return to their own homes. One of them told me that nurses and attendants 'lie' only to soothe them as in reality it would never happen.

Back in the nineteenth century, the district jail at Hazareebagh was converted into a 'lunatic asylum' and the inmates of the jail were sent to the central jail there, which was then newly constructed. The government ordered the removal of almost 250 patients from both the Patna and Berhampore Asylums to the Hazareebagh Asylum. A Committee was appointed to inquire and report the condition of the jail buildings.[150]

In 1876, the Bengal Government, owing to the increasing number of inmates, established the 'lunatic asylum' at Hazareebagh. In an Order,[151] the Government of Bengal complained against the Government of India stating that they

> are not prepared to admit that it is the duty of the state to provide everywhere a certain amount of asylum accommodation sufficient for the assumed lunatic population of the country, irrespective of the fact whether the lunatics themselves are collected by the means which the law provides, or whether proper precautions have been taken to see that the law itself is carefully administered and not stretched to its extreme limits. The tendency among public officers is to admit into asylums, from a spirit of compassion, as many lunatics as the asylum can contain . . .[152]

Therefore, by the time Hazareebagh Lunatic Asylum was established, the administrators had more control over the management of patients and asylums. The rules and regulations set to administer the asylums had also changed. While until the mid-nineteenth century, the consumption of intoxicating substances was considered an important cause of insanity, and anybody found labouring under its influence was sent to the asylum and diagnosed as insane, by 1860s the situation had changed. New rules were set up so as not to accept 'lunatic' persons suffering only from the effects of intoxicating drugs or spirits. Additionally, asylums also refused to admit without payment those patients whose friends were able to compensate for their care. The increase in the number of patients admitted perhaps meant the successful treatment of 'lunacy' during the period, but it also pointed out the inefficiency on the part of the administration—not only did they fail to provide adequate accommodation but the kind of treatment administered was also questionable. Alternatively, to cope with the situation, certain rules were changed. For instance, it was thought of as 'unnecessary' and 'unwise' to admit and maintain all the mentally

[150] Home, Medical, Number 135, Letter from A. Hilson to the Chief Secretary to the Government of Bengal, 8 April, 1890,

[151] Home, Medical Board Proceedings, Number 29, September 1877, NAI.

[152] Home, Medical Board Proceedings, Number 30, September 1877, NAI.

ill persons at a public expense in the government asylums. Hence, entry into the public asylums was restricted to those suffering from 'temporary' effects of sickness, 'intemperance', or 'debauchery', and those whom their friends or family could support. In its initial days, the medical officers considered that a 'lunatic' was better taken care of in an asylum than at the residence, but by the late nineteenth century, this view was no longer prevalent. Instead the government stated that

> many insane are, as a matter of fact, well taken care of by their friends, better indeed and with more tenderness than they can be ordinarily tended at a govt asylum, whereas others, and specially those who are but partially insane and harmless, are best left alone.[153]

The asylum at Hazareebagh was eventually vacated and its inmates were transferred to other institutions.

THE MOYDAPORE LUNATIC ASYLUM

The peripheral location of the Moydapore Asylum made it impossible for 'asylum makers' to exercise a similar degree of supervision over the establishment. 'The fatal objection to the asylum', according to the Lieutenant Governor, 'was its great distance from the Station where the medical officer in charge must necessarily reside'. Because of this distance, the Civil Surgeon regretted that the visits of the ex-officio visitors to the institution who were encouraging to the officials of the establishment, had, as the records in the visiting book showed, been like angels' visits, 'few and far between'.[154] Unlike at the Patna Lunatic Asylum, the asylum at Moydapore was saved from the effects of the great flood of 1861, which inundated the banks of Bhagirathy and Ganges. Many people of Moydapore Asylum fell sick, but the medical officers were able to control the situation.[155]

[153] Home, Medical Board Proceedings, Number 32, September 1877, NAI.

[154] A. Fleming, 'Report on the Moorshedabad Lunatic Asylum for the Year 1862', Officiating Civil Surgeon, Moorshedabad, Superintendent, in *Annual Reports of the Insane Asylums in Bengal for the Years 1862–66* by J. McClleland, Officiating Principal Inspector General, Medical Department (Calcutta: Military Orphan Press, 1863). NAI.

[155] Bengal Proceedings, Medical Department, Number 4, 4 February 1862, APAC, BL.

The Moydapore Asylum was situated in an open plain 4 ¾ miles from the civil and military stations of Berhampore.[156] In 1861, the size of the window opening in each cell was reduced. Those were formerly 4 square feet, and placed on a low footing, which allowed the cold, damp air to pass freely inside the cell. Hence, the lower two feet of these apertures were rebuilt and their width reduced to three feet. Toilet arrangements for the night were also introduced in the corner of each cell, pans were guarded by iron bars supported on pukka masonry, and removed through apertures made in the outer wall. Ventilators were also made in the roof mainly over the privies.[157] The building was designed for an asylum, but by December 1865, the government ordered its total abolition as the building was found unsuitable for further functioning and the inmates were sent to Dullunda and Dacca Asylums. This resulted in the largest population at both of these asylums in 1865. According to A. Fleming, Civil Surgeon, Moorshedabad, the government had abolished the Moydapore Asylum entirely due to financial reasons. He further stated that the decision saved the government from its financial difficulties, but considerably increased the mortality among patients by subjecting them to the hardships of distant travel, such as exposure to cold, heat and rain, and irregular diet.[158]

One reason why this asylum was constructed on the outskirts of the town was because of the increased mortality rate in the Asylum of Calcutta, which according to the medical officers was due to the insalubrious climatic condition there. Hence, 'natives' sent in from the rural districts of Bengal often died by the time they were sent to the centrally located Asylum of Calcutta as they were unaccustomed to the 'foul air and bad water of a crowded metropolis'.[159]

[156] Home Department, Public Proceedings, 19 December 1868, Responses to James Clark's queries on the Moydapore Asylum responded by Surgeon Major A. Fleming, M. D., Civil Surgeon, Moorshedabad, NAI.

[157] Bengal Proceedings, Medical Department, Number 23, 20 February 1861, Report on the Moydapore Lunatic Asylum for the Year 1861 by Surgeon J. Guise, Civil Surgeon Moorshedabad, APAC, BL.

[158] Home Department, Public Proceedings, 19 December 1868, Responses by A. Fleming.

[159] Home Department, Public Proceedings, 19 December 1868, Responses by A. Fleming.

PLAN FOR A CENTRAL LUNATIC ASYLUM

At the close of the nineteenth century, the Government of Bengal was unable to manage so many asylums scattered all over Bengal. A central asylum, they thought, would solve the problem. In a centralized institution, according to the Lieutenant Governor, more attention could be given to the systematic treatment of mental disease than was possible under the existing condition. The government wanted to execute a plan for a central asylum as early as possible.[160]

It was decided that the asylum should be located at Berhampore, which was the most suitable place available in terms of health and convenience, and that only the asylums of Dullunda, Patna, and Berhampore should be combined, leaving the asylums of Bhawanipur, Dacca, and Cuttack outside its fold. The government provisioned special arrangements for the training of civil hospital assistants recruited for government service in the treatment of mental diseases. The government decided to send those qualified physicians immediately on recruitment to asylums to undergo training for two months for the treatment of insanity. It was settled by the asylum administrators that the hospital assistants recruited from the Campbell Medical School at Sealdah, Calcutta and Temple Medical School in Patna would be sent to the Central Asylum at Berhampore, and those recruited from the Dacca and Cuttack schools to the asylums at those places.[161] This illustrated a shift from the usual practice, which was initiated at the beginning of the nineteenth century. It was no longer considered necessary for physicians to be trained in Europe and England. Instead, the medical teachers in schools such as Campbell Medical School, Sealdah, and Temple Medical School, Patna who were formerly trained in England now taught the future medical practitioners.

Throughout the nineteenth century, the medical officers along with the government constantly endeavoured to construct a new asylum or to expand the existing building through necessary construction. This

[160] Home, Medical, August 1896, Letter sent to the Secretary to the Government of India in Home Department from H. Risley, Secretary to the Government of Bengal, NAI.

[161] Home Department, Medical Branch, Number 52, September 1900, 'Annual Report on the Lunatic Asylums of India for 1899,' by E. N. Baker.

thoughtful attempt at last took shape towards the end of the nineteenth century. Construction or additions to the buildings were no longer randomly done. Rather, it was determined by the understanding of the medical practitioners based on the kind of treatment they wanted to provide to the patients. For example, the necessity of solitary confinement as a part of moral treatment made the construction of special cells mandatory even when the problem of overcrowding continued and the asylum managers failed to provide necessary arrangements. They gradually prioritized the issues and made changes accordingly. Barry Edginton had pointed out the connections between architecture and treatment and traced it to nineteenth-century ideas on treatment of insanity, which 'embodied a moral and psychological' view that madness could not be remedied only by kindness but also by a 'proper atmosphere and kindness', which was moral treatment.[162] Therefore, the asylums of the time were constantly built and rebuilt; they went through a series of renovations, additions, and new constructions. The asylum managers often expressed their discontent while choosing a site or making necessary additions to it. As the method of treatment at the asylums by the early nineteenth century was gradually dominated by moral therapy, the medical officers accordingly modified their plans to fit into the criteria of moral treatment.

Several asylums discussed here showed how differences of opinion and the need for new buildings led to the building of asylums during the period. The geographical location of an asylum was one of the most important factors. While the asylums were initially located near water bodies, either river or sea, they slowly shifted to the centre of the town and eventually to the outskirts. Asylums ceased to be the dominant aspect of the cityscape. Instead, inmates were shut within closed walls away from the public eye. It was expected that moral treatment would 'instil in the patient, both physically and mentally, a new set of habits, allowing the patient to become a new person: a sane person'.[163] In the second phase, the shift was due to the necessity felt

[162] Barry Edginton, 'A Space for Moral Management: The York Retreat's Influence on Asylum Design', in *Madness, Architecture and the Built Environment, Psychiatric Spaces in Historical Context*, edited by Leslie Topp, James E. Moran, and Jonathan Andrews (New York: Routledge, 2007), 86.

[163] Edginton, 'A Space for Moral Management', 100.

by the Medical Board to provide a scenic background surrounding the asylum, which was considered as one of the necessary prerequisites of moral treatment. By the close of the nineteenth century, asylum buildings again returned to a central location when the plan for a central mental hospital was proposed. Waterborne diseases and the distance from the town caused the initial shift. Marshy, swampy lands increased physical illnesses, and consequently, it delayed treatment. Besides, most of the medical officers were positioned in the middle of the town or city. Therefore, asylums got shifted to the centre.

Although the intention was to implement the practice in India as it existed in Britain, medical officials faced difficulty in exercising it as the situation was different in the colonial context. This was because government policies differed, and because the superintendents of different asylums differed in their views. Towards the end of the nineteenth century and with the emergence of medical dominance in the treatment of the mentally ill, asylums regained their central locality. This change was due to the understanding of insanity as a disease that could be medically treated. The construction of asylums and their inner arrangements was determined by the method of treatment. Insanity was enclosed within four walls away from the public sphere. However, the architecture continued to be an incessant reminder of the disease and its treatment.

2

TREATMENT OF THE INSANE
CONFLICT BETWEEN THEORY AND PRACTICE

THE TREATMENT PRACTISED IN AN asylum was directly connected with the understanding of insanity and the plan of the asylum. Therefore, this chapter studies the different kinds of treatment practised and their consequences. The therapeutic means adopted in the asylum by the medical officers could be broadly divided into three categories: mechanical, moral, and medical. The moral treatment could further be divided into two: occupational and recreational. Since the turn of the nineteenth century, mechanical restraint, applied with chains, waistcoats, leather jackets, and in many other harsh ways, were questioned in France and elsewhere in Europe by the advocates of moral treatment of insanity such as Pinel, William Tuke, John Haslam, Robert Gardiner, and later John Conolly. Instead of such coercive practices, they put forth notions of moral and humane treatment. In this new method of treatment, mechanical restraint was abolished and shackles were expected to be removed from the patients: a humane mode of treatment was expected to replace the inhumane one. Attendants and medical officers were directly engaged in the treatment. This application of moral therapy involved an engagement with the bodies of the patients as attendants were employed to take physical care of the 'lunatics' for twenty-four hours. Attendants were employed for caring and guarding the patients. Moral therapy was meant to discipline the inmates, without any application of force or coercion.

There was an attempt to implement such practices in the asylums in Bengal. European medical officers made an effort to put an end to the use of chains, waistcoats, leather jackets, and so on, but mechanical restraint could never be completely abolished. The asylum authorities justified the practice of mechanical restraint in certain cases, particularly while dealing with violent and maniac patients. This explained that using any method of coercion in treating the insane was considered easier than medical or moral therapies. Regardless of the attempt to implement moral methods of treatment, restraint continued to be practised in the asylums of Bengal. Moral therapy therefore, did not completely replace mechanical restraints.

Occupational and recreational activities exercised an important role as a part of moral treatment. It was expected that engagement with such activities would have a positive effect on the inmates and help to cure their illness. Medical treatment of 'lunatics' was already in practice even before the idea of an alternative treatment emerged. This chapter demonstrates how far restraint, non-restraint, and medical practices were used in the treatment of the mentally ill in the Lower Provinces of Bengal. In order to do so, it is necessary to examine the stages of development of the different forms of treatment, because their implementation changed the way mental illness was understood in the nineteenth century. For instance, when insanity was understood as a physical disease, medical treatment was practised, but when it was understood as a disease of the mind, then moral treatment was implemented. Physicians, who looked at insanity as both a disease of the mind and body, practised both kinds of treatment.

In the asylums in Bengal, both medical and moral treatments were practised. While medical practitioners used purgatives, sedatives, and tonics to control the initial excitement among patients, the overall healing was based on restraint by moral treatment, which included engagement in various types of asylum labour and certain kinds of amusement as a part of recreation.

Another form of treatment was also known during the period, which H. Van Leeuwen, physician at the asylum in Meerenbergh, North Holland, termed as 'medico-moral treatment'. This required a proper combination of peculiar pharmaceutical, hygienic, moral and social means, fitted to operate on the general bodily health of the insane, and to improve their moral condition by acting upon the feelings, affections, habits, and inclinations.[1]

According to him, it was an anthropological diagnosis where the patient's body was not seen separately as a division between body and soul, but as a unity. The patient was an individual, all his or her physical, intellectual, moral, and social relations should be considered together. He further stated that the medico-moral or anthropological treatment of the insane as opposed to medical treatment constituted the 'true radical indication in every case of insanity'.[2]

The treatment of insanity according to John Bucknill and Daniel Tuke could be hygienic, moral, and medicinal. The removal of a patient from home was hygienic because it removed the patient from the causes of the disease. It was moral, because it produced novel mental impressions and it was medicinal because of the medicine that was necessary for the complete cure.[3]

EVOLUTION OF TREATMENT: MECHANICAL RESTRAINT TO MORAL THERAPY

Before discussing the methods of treatment, it is necessary to trace the evolution of treatment from mechanical to moral therapy and to trace the engagement between the two. European physicians were in charge of the asylums in Bengal throughout the nineteenth century. In order to understand what made them implement mechanical or non-mechanical restraint in these asylums, it is necessary to trace the path through which they travelled; physicians studied medicine back

[1] H. Van Leeuwen, 'On the Medico and Moral Treatment of Insanity,' *Asylum Journal of Mental Sciences*, no. 6 (1 July 1854): 91–3, Association of Medical Officers of Asylums and Hospitals for the Insane, London, 1855, Wellcome Library for the History of Medicine [henceforth WL].

[2] Van Leeuwen, 'On the Medico and Moral Treatment of Insanity,' 91–3.

[3] John Charles Bucknill and Daniel Hack Tuke, *A Manual of Psychological Medicine: Containing the History, Nosology, Description, Statistics, Diagnosis, Pathology and Treatment of Insanity, with an Appendix of Cases* (London: John Churchill, 1862), 498, WL.

at home, practised it, and, at the same time, implemented it in the colonies. This journey also explains why mechanical restraint could never be completely removed from the asylums in colonial Bengal even after the acceptance of moral therapy as a humane mode of treatment by the medical officers. Mechanical restraint was not completely abolished and the 'moral managers' continued its use on the pretext that it was necessary to control violent patients in order to save them from injuring themselves or others.

In 1791 and 1792 two important books on the practice of non-mechanical restraint in French asylums were published by two noted medical practitioners. In England, the practice was implemented in asylums much before 1791, but it gained popularity only after William Tuke started its practice in the Retreat Asylum. Philippe Pinel (1745–1826) of France was well known as one of the first proponents who advocated the practice of non-restraint in the asylum. By 1792, he liberated fifty-three patients confined in Bicétre from chains[4] and thereby paved the path for moral and humane treatment. Pinel's historic act became so popular that another man, who also had tried to implement moral therapy even before Pinel's time, was overlooked. In the year 1791, a French physician at Chambéry named M. Daguin (1732–1815), in his book *On the Philosophy of Madness* pointed out that this malady ought to be treated by moral rather than by physical means.[5] In this book, he advocated the abolition of the imprisonment of the insane in cells and their coercion by chains. He proposed that inmates should be allowed a greater degree of freedom in a spacious and pleasant enclosure where they should be able to wander at will. Daguin, who admired Pinel, realized even before the latter that mentally ill people needed treatment and not just incarceration.[6] John Bucknill criticized Pinel whose name was 'canonised in the records

---

[4] Bucknill and Tuke, *A Manual of Psychological Medicine*, 52.

[5] M. Daguin, *On the Philosophy of Madness* (Chambéry: Gorrin, 1791).

[6] John Bucknill made these comments while reviewing Daniel Hack Tuke's book. John Bucknill, 'The Progressive Changes which Have Taken Place since the Time of Pinel in the Moral Management of the Insane, and the Various Contrivances which have been Adopted Instead of Mechanical Restraint', *The Asylum Journal of Mental Science*, Association of Medical Officers of Asylums and Hospitals for the Insane, no. 9, (15 November 1854): 157, WL.

of mental science'. Pinel, who had acknowledged many authors of his own times and of the past when he published *Medico Philosophical Treatise on Mania* in 1801, remained completely silent about Daguin, whereas Daguin dedicated the second edition of his book to Pinel.[7]

By narrating this Bucknill not only tried to prove that Pinel's supremacy as the first proponent of moral treatment could be questioned, but by tracing the lineage of moral treatment in England he also tried to establish the supremacy of English physicians over French and thereby exposed the rivalry therein.

The history of the humane treatment of the insane and the origin of what is called the non-restraint system, according to John Bucknill, started in England. It began with the establishment of Bethlem Hospital for mentally ill patients in 1675. In the rules made for its functioning in 1677 it was stated that 'lunatics' should be permitted to walk in the yard until dinner time, following which they would be locked up in their cells.[8] Bucknill further said that

> no lunatic that lies naked, or is in a course of physic, should be seen by the physician without an order of the physician. It is further humanely ordered, that no officer or servant shall beat or abuse any lunatic, nor employ any force to them, but upon absolute necessity for the better governing of them.[9]

In order to establish the supremacy of the English physicians over the French, Bucknill made a detailed list of books written by English physicians. H. M. Herwig published *Art of Curing Sympathetically or Magnetically; with a Discourse on the Cure of Madness* in 1700; in 1705 Thomas Fallowes enlightened the world with his *Method of Curing Lunatics*; Robert Blakeway wrote *An Essay Towards the Cure of Religious Melancholy: in a Letter to a Gentlewoman Afflicted with it* in 1717; followed by *A Treatise on Phrensy* by P. Frings in 1746 and *Treatise on Madness* by Batty in 1757. But, according to Bucknill, none of their works gained enough reputation. In 1789, Harper's *A Treatise on the Real Cause and Cure of Insanity* was criticized by Pinel. In 1790, *Observations on the General and Improper Treatment of Insanity* by Faulkner was

[7] Bucknill, 'Progressive Changes since the Time of Pinel,' 157.

[8] Bucknill and Tuke, *A Manual of Psychological Medicine*, 53.

[9] Bucknill and Tuke, *A Manual of Psychological Medicine*, 53.

published and the *Observations on Maniacal Disorders* was published by Pargeter in 1792.[10]

It seemed as if none of these treatises could help ameliorate the condition of the lunatics in the asylums of England, until William Tuke established the York Retreat and implemented methods of non-restraint there.[11] According to Dr Thurnam,

> it was in the spring of 1792, the very year in which the celebrated Pinel commenced the amelioration of the treatment of the insane in France, by the truly courageous act of unchaining fifty supposed incurable and dangerous lunatics at the Bicêtre, that the establishment of the Retreat (at York) was proposed by the late William Tuke.[12]

John Conolly commented on the practice of restraint in the Retreat:

> Restraint was not altogether abolished by them (the early managers of the Retreat), but they undoubtedly began the new system of treatment in this country, and the restraints they did continue to resort to were of the mildest kind.[13]

According to John Bucknill, other than the difference in the practice of restraint in France and in England, one major difference between the physicians of these two countries was that while the former did not praise their predecessors, the latter had always been thankful and full of appreciation in such terms as 'to prove him a single minded advocate for the insane, forgetful of his own claims in the earnestness

---

[10] See H. M. Herwig, *Art of Curing Sympathetically or Magnetically; With a Discourse on the Cure of Madness* (London: Tho. Newborough, 1700); Thomas Fallowes, *Method of Curing Lunatics* (London: For the Author, 1705); Robert Blakeway, *An Essay Towards the Cure of Religious Melancholy: In a Letter to a Gentlewoman Afflicted with It* (London: Bezaleel Creake, 1717); P. Frings, *A Treatise on Phrensy* (London: T. Gardner, 1746); William Battie, *Treatise on Madness* (London: Whiston and White, 1757); Andrew Harper, *A Treatise on the Real Cause and Cure of Insanity* (London: Stalker 1789); Benjamin Faulkner, *Observations on the General and Improper Treatment of Insanity* (London: Reynell, 1789); and William Pargeter, *Observations on Maniacal Disorders* (Reading: For the Author, 1792).

[11] Bucknill and Tuke, *A Manual of Psychological Medicine*, 53.

[12] Bucknill and Tuke, *A Manual of Psychological Medicine*, 56.

[13] Bucknill and Tuke, *A Manual of Psychological Medicine*, 58.

of his demands for them'.[14] Daniel Tuke had pointed out that French physicians used seclusion in addition to restraint, such as the use of a waistcoat, whereas the English only used the latter. The *cellule* (cell) of a Parisian asylum was usually a single-bedded room, while in England solitary cells were usually empty and carefully guarded padded rooms. Therefore, it was one thing to leave a violent patient with suicidal tendencies alone in a non-padded roomv and another to leave him in a padded room, because in case of the latter the chance of injuries by running his or her head against the wall were non-existent. Therefore, an inmate in a padded room was considered safer in comparison to one in a non-padded room as in France.

In India, padded rooms were difficult to maintain. According to the Superintendent of the Dacca Lunatic Asylum, instead of padded rooms, the asylum had two cells for solitary confinement. The climatic condition of eastern India was not conducive for padded rooms, because the presence of white ants often proved to be disastrous as they usually destroyed the pads.[15] This problem continued even at the end of the century as pestilent measures were yet to establish their own footing. Therefore, an addition was thought of along with the pads, which, it was hoped, would improve the situation. Hence, at the Patna Lunatic Asylum, padded cells were covered with canvas from the inside. But they started rotting because of humidity immediately after their application and were considered useless.[16] Therefore, the practice of confinement of mentally ill patients in padded cells was not much of a success in India.

From Pinel to Conolly, there were lots of debates on the abolition of mechanical restraints in the asylums of Europe and England and about their applications. An attempt was made to replace mechanical restraint with moral treatment, thereby providing the space for the gradual formation of a new method of treatment. Roy Porter had termed it

[14] Bucknill, 'Progressive Changes since the Time of Pinel,' 159.

[15] Home Department, Public Proceedings, 19 December 1868, Letter from James Wise, Superintendent of Lunatic Asylums, Dacca to William Keates, Deputy Inspector General of Hospitals, Dacca Circle, dated 24 June 1868, NAI.

[16] Municipal Department, Medical Branch, Number 5801, 26 April 1898, Remarks made by Colonel T. H. Hendeley, I. M. S., Inspector General of Civil Hospitals, Bengal, on the Patna Lunatic Asylum, 24 November 1898, NAI.

'moral management'.[17] According to him, it was 'moral' because it addressed the patients' mind rather than the body and 'management' as the 'mad doctor had to prove consummately dynamic and resourceful, prolific in initiatives designed to impose discipline and sanity'.[18]

In Bengal's asylums, there was an attempt to abolish such practices, although it was not wholly implemented. Moral and medical therapy continued to be practised along with mechanical restraints in asylums. The decisions of the Commissioners in Lunacy in England were frequently followed and practised by the Bengal medical practitioners. The Commissioners in Lunacy in their Report to the Lord Chancellor in 1847 stated that

> moral treatment of insanity comprehends all those means which, by operating on the feelings and habits, exert a salutary influence, and tend to restore thee, to a sound and natural state.[19]

Moral treatment in the late eighteenth and nineteenth centuries was understood as a mild, humane treatment without restraints, which was 'a concentration on the rational and emotional rather than the organic causes of insanity'.[20] The asylum medical practitioners claimed that they carefully dealt with the demands and complaints of the patients with kindness, sympathy, and attention in order to get their confidence and also to contribute to their comfort and well-being. The point principally in view of those practitioners was to teach patients discipline and habits of self-control. In their reports, they often stated that harsh methods of punishment were not necessary and personal restraint was seldom resorted to. However, confinement in solitary cells was a form of harsh treatment, which was probably equivalent to or more traumatic than other kinds of severe punishment by physical restraints. For instance, during the day time, the inmates were at liberty to move about freely

[17] Roy Porter, 'Shaping Psychiatric Knowledge: The Role of the Asylum,' in *Medicine in the Enlightenment* (Amsterdam and Atlanta, GA: Rodopi, 1995), 255–73, WL.

[18] Porter, 'Shaping Psychiatric Knowledge,' 255–73.

[19] Van Leeuwen, 'On the Medico and Moral Treatment of Insanity,' 91–93.

[20] Anne Digby, 'Moral Treatment at the Retreat,' in *The Anatomy of Madness*, Vol. 2, edited by W. F. Bynum, R. Porter, and M. Shepard (London: Tavistock, 1985), 53, WL.

within the compound of the asylum. However, when anyone was found guilty of unruly conduct or had quarrels with other patients, he or she was confined in seclusion in the cell for the entire day or perhaps only for a few hours, until the inmate gave in to 'professed penitence and promised good behaviour'.[21]

The Superintendent of the Moorshedabad Asylum in the Berhampore district of Bengal took recourse to restraint as well as to medical treatment, as he found both necessary for the treatment of the mentally ill. For instance, leather belts were used to tie 'lunatics' prior to the superintendence of Alexander Russell, who replaced them with cotton tapes, as leather got hard in the tropical climate. The use of iron fetters was also justified by the superintendent on the pretext that lack of space kept all the cells occupied. Thus, those patients who were placed in the corridors were chained so that they could not do any harm to themselves or to others. According to the superintendent, an increase in the number of cells would help to avoid such harsh treatment.[22] But the increase in cells meant an increase in solitary confinement rather than the use of chains or probably both were practiced in a solitary dark room. Solitary confinement was no less serious a punishment than tying the inmates in chains. Patients were at times confined in those cells for hours, and at times, for a few days in continuation.

Even a proponent of moral treatment like Daniel Tuke clearly stated his opinion in *Moral Management of the Insane*, both in favour and against mechanical restraint, as he practised both for treating his patients at the York Retreat. According to him, reasons why mechanical restraint should not be used in an asylum were, first, that non-restraint was the most humane and less irritating mode of treatment. At the same time, it also encouraged and strengthened the self-control of the patient. Second, recovery under such circumstances was likely to be permanent. Third, mechanical restraint degraded the mind because of its bad moral

[21] Medical Board Proceedings, May 1842, Report submitted to W. Findon, Superintending Surgeon, Presidency Division, on the State of the Insane Hospital at Moorshedabad by A. Kean, Civil Assistant Surgeon, Moorshedabad, 26 March 1842, NAI.

[22] Medical Board Proceedings, Number 39, 11 June 1821, Letter from Russell, Superintending Surgeon, Berhampore to James Jameson, Secretary to the Medical Board Calcutta, dated 25 May 1821, NAI.

effect. Fourth, prior experience demonstrated that there was more tranquillity in those asylums where this system (non-restraint) was adopted; lastly, mechanical restraint was liable to great abuse from the keepers. At the same time, his argument in favour of mechanical restraint was that it was necessary to acquire quicker authority over the patients. Second, although authority might be obtained in a majority of cases by persuasion, there were also instances when it failed. Third, mechanical restraint completely prevented injury to the patients or to others. Fourth, attendants were not to be trusted in their manual restraint of patients. Fifth, mechanical restraint was less irritating than manual treatment. Sixth, it reduced the cost of extra attendants, which was otherwise difficult to maintain in the poorer asylums of England. Seventh, exercise in the open air was compatible with mechanical restraint unlike seclusion in single rooms. Eighth, the practice of seclusion was essentially coercive, which was objected to on moral grounds. Lastly, he concluded from his experiences that mechanical restraint was necessary.[23] Therefore, moral treatment along with mechanical restraint was considered to be a humane treatment for the 'lunatics'. Both the practices overlapped as the advocates of moral treatment could not clearly demarcate the boundaries of their practices. While they criticized mechanical restraint, they themselves partly took recourse to it as well.

Degrees of insanity determined the kind of treatment practised. A member of the Medical Board, J. Swiney, stated in 1835 that there were less incidents of mania in India than in Europe. Therefore, according to him, it was seldom necessary to put the Indian patients in solitary confinement or use straitjackets. Violent cases were less prevalent among Bengalis than among up-countrymen. The most common form of insanity in India, according to J. Swiney, was 'eccentric mania'. He further stated that there was more of 'passive imbecility than of raving madness among the Bengalis'.[24] In 1842, inmates at the Dacca

---

[23] Daniel Tuke, *Moral Management of the Insane and the Various Contrivances which have been Adopted Instead of Mechanical Restraint* (London: John Churchill, 1854), 84–85, WL.

[24] Medical Board Proceedings, Number 8, 26 March 1835, Letter sent to James Hutchinson, Secretary to Medical Board from J. Swiney, Second Member in Charge of Superintendent Surgeon Office Presidency, dated 24 March 1835, NAI.

Lunatic Asylum were put in solitary cells whenever they could not be controlled. Other than such confinements, straitjackets were also used. According to the Civil Surgeon of Dacca, 'native' insane patients were easily managed and controlled by putting them in solitary cells and using straitjackets.[25] The Superintendent of the Dacca Asylum James Wise stated that in the period between 1850 and 1851, manacles were tied around the feet and hands of dangerous 'lunatics'. He further stated that since 1853 mechanical restraint was not practised at the Dacca Asylum. The application of mechanical coercion, according to him, was eventually replaced by solitary confinement. Confinement in a solitary cell for a few hours, curtailing the daily allowance of tobacco, or prohibiting their recreational activities were also considered by medical officers as efficient punishment for mischievous and unmanageable patients instead of putting them in chains.[26]

Different forms of restraint continued in the asylums of Bengal even after the superintendents were aware of its misuses. By the year 1870, 'woollen bag' was used to restrain patients in the Dullunda Asylum. The Superintendent of the asylum wrote in the Annual Report that its usage was not only confined to restrict inmates from hurting themselves or their neighbours, but also to control excitements when no other sort of treatment could help. He further stated that such a practice restrained mischievous movements without causing discomfort or alarm to the patient. It was more 'gentle', 'safe', and 'strong' than the hands of the best tempered attendants, and thus effectively prevented one principal cause of fatal exhaustion in patients suffering from any sort of mania. However, the death of a violent 'lunatic' due to the use of 'woollen bag' finally forced him to stop such practice in the asylum.[27] The mode of restraint practised at Dullunda Asylum in

[25] Medical Board Proceedings, May 1842, Letter sent to Robert Brown, Officiating Surgeon from J. Taylor, Civil Surgeon Dacca, dated 2 May 1842, NAI.

[26] Home Department, Public Proceedings, Letter from James Wise to William Keates, 24 June 1868.

[27] *General Report Number 3 on the Lunatic Asylums, Vaccinations and Dispensaries in the Bengal Presidency for the Year 1870*, compiled by Assistant Surgeon K. McLeod, Officiating Secretary to the Inspector General of Hospitals, Indian Medical Department (Calcutta: Bengal Secretariat Press, 1872), NAI.

1871 was a belt, which was fastened round the wrist with a short chain and with handcuffs on each side.[28] The medical officers were bound to mention the usage of various forms of restraints in the asylums in their reports. Such usage was already considered harmful by the practitioners in England. Therefore, the medical practitioners in India also stated towards the end of their reports that even though the option of such practices did exist here, yet, usually the officers often did not take recourse to them.

Samuel Tuke's *Description of the Retreat*[29] published in 1813 suggested the replacement of the old general treatments of insanity, bloodletting, blisters, setons,[30] evacuants, and many other prescriptions of physical coercion with moral therapy. Instead, it consisted of a regime that included nutritious diet, frequent exercise, fresh air, and hot- and cold-water baths. The purpose was to maintain physical well-being, orderliness, and relaxation amongst the patients. According to Daniel Hack Tuke, moral treatment was based on kindness in contrast to earlier methods of inhumane treatment. It was a method in which 'moral principles were carved upon the very foundation stone of the building'.[31] Moral therapy necessitated a new kind of asylum architecture, one that could be used as a form of treatment in itself rather than a method which would facilitate the treatment.

Robert Gardiner Hill, member of the Royal College of Surgeons and Resident Medical Superintendent of the Lincolnshire County Asylum, stated that in a properly constructed building with a sufficient number of suitable attendants, the total abolition of mechanical restraint was both practicable and humane. He advocated careful vigilance by attendants, a suitable planning of the building, and particularly moral treatment,

[28] Superintendent B. Simpson, 'Report on the Patna Lunatic Asylum for the Year 1871,' in *Annual Report on Insane Asylums of Bengal for the Year 1871* by J. Campbell Brown, Inspector General of Hospitals, Indian Medical Department (Calcutta: Bengal Secretariat Press, 1872), NAI.

[29] Samuel Tuke, *Description of the Retreat* ([1813]; reprint, London: Process Press, 1996).

[30] A skein of cotton, or similar material, passed below the skin and left with the ends protruding to promote drainage, and such like.

[31] For further details on Daniel Hack Tuke's writings, see Edginton, 'A Space for Moral Management', 87.

which, according to him, would help to induce habits of self-control in the patients. He further believed that restraint could not be completely abolished. Therefore, instead of putting fetters on the inmates or using any other form of severe bodily torture, he suggested that in the case of maniac patients and inmates during their paroxysms of violence, the most 'simple means should be selected', which meant seclusion in a dark room.[32] On the issue of seclusion, the Eighth Commissioner in Lunacy in his report issued in 1854 stated that

> its occasional use is generally considered beneficial. Its employment by harsh or indolent persons is liable of great abuse, and that it should only be employed with the knowledge and direct sanction of the medical officer.[33]

Handcuffs were used in the Moydapore Asylum, although according to A. Fleming, Civil Surgeon at Moorshedabad Asylum, its usage was rare. Handcuffs were not kept in the asylum but usually borrowed from the nearby jail. It was used to control violent patients who often tried to destroy the masonry work of their cells.[34] This showed that the medical officers did not often differentiate between the practice of restraint on a jail inmate and on an inmate in an asylum as both institutions were looked upon by them as a prison where correctional methods were applied. Interestingly, although the type of inmates taken into confinement differed, the treatment was similar in most of the instances.

[32] Robert Gardiner Hill, *A Concise History of the Entire Abolition of Mechanical Restraint in the Treatment of the Insane; and of the Introduction, Success, and Final Triumph of the Non Restraint System, Together with a Reprint of a Lecture Delivered on the Subject in the Year 1838 and Appendices, Containing an Account of the Controversies and Claims Connected Therewith* (London: Longman, Brown, Green, and Longmans, Paternoster Row, 1857), WL.

[33] John Charles Bucknill (ed.), *Asylum Journal of Mental Sciences*, Number 8, 1 October 1854, (London: Association of Medical Officers of Asylums and Hospitals for the Insane, 1855): 113–15, WL.

[34] Home Department, Public Proceedings, 19 December 1868, From Surgeon Major A. Fleming, Civil Surgeon, Moorshedabad, to the Deputy Inspector General of Hospitals, Presidency Division, Calcutta, Number 21, Berhampore, dated 15 July 1868, NAI. This was sent as a reply to Sir James Clark's questions regarding the cure and treatment of lunatics in India.

Restraint continued to be practised in the Dullunda and Patna Asylums by means of ligatures,[35] bags, belts, chains, and handcuffs. The superintendents of both the asylums justified the usage of such restraints only in instances where it was necessary to prevent the patient from meddling with his sores or wounds.[36] However, according to J. Campbell Brown, its adoption as an asylum practice inculcated and maintained among attendants an entirely false and wrong notion as to how inmates should be treated. He further stated that it was impossible to dissociate the idea of coercion or punishment from the imposition of restraint. Hence, according to him, the imposition of manual restraint was by no means a necessary alternative, and was seldom found in asylums where the idea and practice of restraint had been abolished.[37] According to the Surgeon Major A. Payne of the Dullunda Asylum, the number of 'lunatics' confined in separate rooms and 'restrained in gentle and beneficial manner' was higher in 1871 than in previous years. The growing experience of the use of woollen bags in cases of violent and frenzied patients made the medical practitioners of the asylums believe that a very mischievous or troublesome inmate was safer alone than in the custody of a 'native' warder outside. According to A. Payne, a 'maniac' dangerous to himself fared much worse under the manual efforts of an attendant than he did when lying in a loose soft bag in an open veranda.[38]

Accidents and injuries increased in the asylum.[39] Although in their reports superintendents did not explain the cause and kind of such

[35] Something that is used to bind, specifically, a filament (as a thread) used in surgery.

[36] Bengal Proceedings, Medical Department, Number 21, 4 October 1872, Letter sent to the Officiating Secretary to the Government of Bengal from J. Campbell Brown, Inspector General of Hospitals, Indian Medical Department, Fort William, dated 27 June 1872, APAC, BL.

[37] *Annual Report on the Insane Asylums in Bengal for the year 1871*, by J. Campbell Brown, Inspector General of Hospitals, Indian Medical Department (Calcutta: Bengal Secretariat Press, 1872), NAI.

[38] A. Payne, 'Report on the Dullunda Asylum for 1871,' *Annual Report on the Insane Asylums in Bengal for the Year 1871.*

[39] Bengal Proceedings, Medical Department, Number 21, 4 October 1871, 'Report on the Dullunda Lunatic Asylum for the Year 1871,' by A. Payne, Superintendent of the Asylum, APAC, BL.

occurrences, it could be assumed that the application of mechanical restraints caused these injuries and accidents amongst the inmates. Attendants were employed to take care of patients and act as a substitute for mechanical restraint. For certain reasons medical officers could not completely rely on them. The acts of medical officers were also questionable. For instance, at the Patna Lunatic Asylum in 1872, Superintendent B. Simpson stated that restraint was used on a patient whose finger had to be amputated on account of a bad sore.[40] The reason that led to such an incident was questionable. The sore on the inmate's finger could have been due to application of harsh restraint. This shows that not only were attendants responsible for the patients' accidents and injuries, but also that the negligence of medical officers often led to such incidents.

There were many advocates of mechanical restraint in the nineteenth century, particularly among French and German physicians, who asserted that cases might arise where the application of mechanical restraint could be imperative. Sir John Bucknill, although one of them, stated that

> mechanical restraint in the treatment of the insane is like the actual cautery in the treatment of wounds, a barbarous remedy, which has become obsolete from the introduction of more skilful and humane methods.[41]

While Bucknill adopted the method of non-restraint, he also believed in the occasional treatment of inmates by the application of restraints. He emphasized the importance of mechanical restraint, particularly during surgical cases. He observed that whether 'sane' or insane, such practices were necessary to ensure the absolute stillness of bodily functions, which was essential for the healing process. But, such practices, according to Hill, could have endangered the life of many.[42]

---

[40] B. Simpson, Surgeon of the Asylum, 'Report on the Patna Lunatic Asylum for the Year 1872,' *Annual Report on the Insane Asylums of Bengal for the Year 1872.*

[41] Robert Gardiner Hill, 'On the Non Restraint System', in *Asylum Journal of Mental Sciences* edited by John Bucknill, Number 10, January 1855 (London: Association of Medical Officers of Asylums and Hospitals for the Insane, 1855), 153–5, WL.

[42] Hill, 'On the Non Restraint System,' 153–5.

A new experiment was implemented in treating the lunatics without restraint in the Patna Lunatic Asylum in 1858 by J. Sutherland, Civil Surgeon. This was suggested by the Superintendent Surgeon, Dr John Balfour. He recommended that only violent and dangerous patients should be locked up, whereas others should be kept in the ward without locking the doors.[43] The medical officers were satisfied with the results. Therefore, this practice continued at the Patna Asylum till the end of the century. According to G. Saunders, Deputy Inspector General of Hospitals, Dinapore Circle, handcuffs, straitjackets, and fixed chairs were not used in the Patna Lunatic Asylum from 1868. Although no separate cells were constructed for confinement, over-excited patients were locked up in a cell for two to three days continuously.[44] According to the Superintendent of the Dacca Lunatic Asylum, mechanical restraint was not in use in the asylum since 1841 other than the occasional use of feet and hand irons during 1851–3.[45] It was evident from what he said that the feet and hand irons were not considered by him as a form of mechanical restraint. In 1841, according to Dr Taylor:

> The strait jacket was rarely applied, and is seldom necessary, indeed, for more than a few hours at a time. There is not a fixed iron ring or chain for restraint in any part of the Asylum; nor have any of the patients, with the exception of the criminal ones, any rings or fetters on their arms or legs.[46]

Waltraud Ernst had pointed out a very significant aspect regarding the application of mechanical restraint in the European Lunatic Asylum of Bengal. According to her, the issue of race and class played a significant role in the application of mechanical restraint. She illustrated how certain

[43] Bengal Proceedings, Medical Department, Number 5, 6 July 1860, 'Report on the Patna Lunatic Asylum for the Year 1859,' by J. Sutherland, Civil Surgeon, Patna, APAC, BL.

[44] Home Department, Public Proceedings, 19 December 1868, Memorandum from G. Saunders, M. D., Deputy Inspector General of Hospitals, Lower Provinces, Number 809, Dinajpore, dated 5 June 1868, forwarded for the information of the Inspector General of Hospital, with reference to his Office Circular Number 13 of the 14 Ultimo, NAI.

[45] Home Department, Public Proceedings, Letter from James Wise to William Keates, 24 June 1868.

[46] Home Department, Public Proceedings, Letter from James Wise to William Keates, 24 June 1868.

classes of soldiers and sailors admitted at the asylum felt humiliated or degraded when they were put under the control of 'native' attendants. Therefore, while the upper-class Europeans of the asylum were taken care of by European attendants, the European lower class or the 'pauper lunatics' were usually looked after by the Indian staff. This was a cause of disgrace for the European 'pauper lunatics' who preferred the use of chains and fetters over being 'mishandled' by 'natives'. This exemplified the hatred of the Europeans towards the 'natives' to the extent that at a time when there were debates on abolishing mechanical restraint, Europeans thought it a better substitute than being 'subdued' by 'native' attendants.[47]

In the 'native' asylums, where there was no class division, and given that the 'natives' were left with no choice of their own to decide on an alternative, moral treatment was probably a milder substitute for the harsh coercive practices of mechanical restraint, although the former was no less traumatic. The dilemma remained in implementing it in practice: the medical officers desired to abolish the application of mechanical restraint, but they could not give it up wholly. This was because they always considered mechanical restraint an easier alternative, particularly while managing violent patients. The officers could not think of an alternative way of treating such inmates. Thus, while certain means of mechanical control were abolished, the idea of restraint continued. Earlier, this was done through the application of certain instruments, but subsequently it was practised by the asylum staff or through solitary confinement in cells. For instance, H. Cayley of the Cuttack Lunatic Asylum stated that cases occasionally occurred where it was realized that a simple form of restraint was less irritating than the forcible holding down of a violent patient. As this was accepted in England,[48] he continued with its practice in India. Often this was the procedure for treatment practised by European medical physicians; they implemented their theory into practice in the colony as a part of their 'civilizing mission'. The hypothesis that such practices might bring similar or

[47] Waltraud Ernst, 'Idioms of Madness and Colonial Boundaries: The Case of the European and "Native" Mentally Ill in Early Nineteenth-Century British India,' *Comparative Studies in Society and History*, vol. 39, no. 1 (January 1997): 153–81.

[48] H. Cayley, 'Report on Cuttack Lunatic Asylum for the Year 1872,' *Annual Report on the Insane Asylums of Bengal for the Year 1872*.

superior results often boomeranged. The problem with this was that due to difference in climatic condition, habits, and ways of everyday living, a practice followed in European continents or in England was not necessarily successful in the case of India or Britain's other colonies.

MEDICAL TREATMENT

The medical practitioners recognized that by the latter half of mid-nineteenth century, only mechanical and moral forms of treatment were not enough for the cure of mentally ill persons. During the earlier period, some of the practitioners tried to implement medical therapies, but the practice discontinued as moral therapy dominated the practice of the day. In this context, Andrew Scull stated that the engagement of 'mad doctors' in the treatment could be traced back to the eighteenth century when moral treatment was not practised in the asylums. The English medical profession at that time was composed of physicians, surgeons, and apothecaries, and each one of them served a different clientele.[49] According to him, the English physicians were the doctors of the elite who generally possessed a medical degree and were also members of the Royal College of Physicians. Only a medical physician (M. D.) had no clinical experience other than an acquaintanceship in the subject with 'classical authors' and was trained at Oxbridge or in similar establishments. Their membership of the College depended more on social networks than on medical sciences. Scull further stated that as 'surgeons had only recently severed their connection with the barber's trade', their status was lower than that of the physicians and their entrance into the ranks of physicians was usually through apprenticeship. Apothecaries were also 'recruited by apprenticeship and lacked control over licensing and entry'.[50] They catered largely to the middle and lower classes. Apothecaries varied from semi-illiterate quacks to highly competent practitioners by the standards of the time.[51] The doctors entering the 'mad business' were not drawn from any of these three classes. Instead, they were from the most educated and literate sections of the profession.

[49] Andrew Scull, *The Most Solitary of Afflictions: Madness and Society in Britain 1700–1900* (New Haven and London: Yale University Press, 1993), 181.

[50] Scull, *The Most Solitary of Afflictions*, 181.

[51] Scull, *The Most Solitary of Afflictions*, 181.

They were amongst the most 'vigorous and effective partisans of medicine's claim in this area', and contributed most to its 'growing dominance of the field'.[52] The eighteenth-century medical practices usually involved purges, vomits, bleedings, and the use of various mysterious coloured powders, whose secrets, Scull claimed, were known only to the compounders who worked under the guidance of the practitioners. With the body viewed as a whole where the organs were interconnected and 'equally capable of affecting each other', doctors justified their claims to the cure of insanity, as a disease of the mind or brain, with their treatments of 'purges, vomits, and bleedings'.[53]

By the beginning of the nineteenth century, medical practitioners were faced with hindrances in their practice due to the emergence of moral treatment. The moral treatment was a non-medical, therapeutic means of treatment. Bloodlettings and other cathartics used by the medical practitioners for treating the patients were questioned by the moral therapists who viewed those practices as embedded in the classical period.[54] Therefore, all these made the position of the medical practitioners vulnerable for some time. As William Bynum put it, with the establishment of the moral therapy at the Retreat, there was 'a rather damning attack on the medical profession's capacity to deal with mental illnesses'.[55] He further pointed out:

> At the Retreat, like the Bicêtre, the physician was a shadowy figure, the burden of therapeutic responsibility having fallen on the keepers and other staff whose personal contacts with the patient were much greater than that of the physician.[56]

Henceforth, physicians' duties were confined to the treatment of physical illness of the 'lunatics' in asylums while attendants were placed in charge of the day-to-day governance of the institution. The 1815–16 Report of the Select Committee on Madhouses provided support for William Tuke's contention that very little could be done by medical

---

[52] Scull, *The Most Solitary of Afflictions*, 182.

[53] Scull, *The Most Solitary of Afflictions*, 183.

[54] Scull, *The Most Solitary of Afflictions*, 185.

[55] William Bynum, 'Rationales for Therapy in British Psychiatry, 1780–1835,' *Medical History* 18 (1964): 323, WL.

[56] Bynum, 'Rationales for Therapy in British Psychiatry', 324.

treatment in cases of mental derangement. Therefore, for many, who had previously disapproved of 'lunacy reforms' on humanitarian grounds, and, according to Scull, 'who had previously lacked a viable alternative to existing asylums', now yielded to moral treatment.[57]

But the medical practitioners who believed mental illness could be cured by medicine did not give up. In 1841 they established the Association of Medical Officers of Asylums and Hospitals for Insane in England. Finally, by 1845, after a prolonged struggle, they could establish the fact that insanity was a disease, which implied that doctors alone were qualified to treat the 'lunatics'. In 1853, the Society started publishing its own periodical named *Asylum Journal*, under the editorship of John Charles Bucknill. Bucknill pointed out that this, along with another journal known as *Journal of Psychological Medicine and Mental Pathology*, edited by Dr Forbes Winslow, published a large number of articles and monographs on the medical treatments of insanity. The publishing of this journal, Bucknill claimed, made it difficult for others to avoid concluding that mental illness could also be treated by medical treatment.

It is within this context that the medical treatment of insanity in the asylums of Bengal is studied. In the context of India, there was also a distinct change in the process of treatment before and after 1858. In the period before 1858, medical treatment was found more useful for the treatment of inmates while the period after reacted with mixed opinions. While the medical practitioners could not overlook the importance of medical treatment, they could also not ignore the effects of moral treatment.

According to G. Lamb, the Civil Surgeon of Dacca Asylum, treatment of mental illness was a difficult procedure because in most of the cases patients were admitted to the asylums without a prior case history. Therefore, it was not possible to know whether it was their first attack or a 'confirmed and hopeless case of long duration'.[58] The Surgeon considered the pathology of the diseases of the brain to be connected with the symptoms of insanity; hence, medical treatment was important for the cure of the inmates, but at the same time, he was also in favour of moral therapy which included exercises and other occupational therapies.

[57] Scull, *The Most Solitary of Afflictions*, 192.
[58] Medical Board Proceedings, Number 7, 9 November 1835, Letter sent to James Hutchinson, Secretary to Medical Board from G. Lamb, Civil Surgeon Dacca, dated 31 October 1835, NAI.

Once a patient was admitted to the asylum, the Surgeon began the treatment by administering purgatives, which he thought would keep the patient quiet for a short time. An initial treatment of this kind, according to Lamb, would give the patient the time to get accustomed to the place and to the confinement, following which the patient entered a detailed course of medical treatment. He practised bloodletting by the application of leeches. According to him, the 'most effectual means of subsiding delirium with actual determination of blood was by the application of cold water on the head allowed to fall from a continuous stream of water'.[59] Heavy dosage of tartar emetic often caused nausea in patients. Blisters were applied on neck and head; it was known to relieve deeper irritation. He found the application of blisters on the abdomen effective, particularly in winter.[60] Other than all of these practices, he considered 'darkness' as an effective sedative for treating insanity, because according to him, patients were usually more noisy on moonlit nights. The effect of the moon was considered an important cause of mental illness during the nineteenth century. According to the Superintendent of the Dacca Lunatic Asylum, 'paroxysms of mental excitement' generally recurred with lunar cycles, and the effect rarely continued for more than a few days. It was noted that a few of the patients under its influence either attempted to strike out at others or were inclined to cause injury to themselves. The violence they committed while 'running amuck' included tearing off their clothes and blankets, pulling out bricks from the walls and shaking the doors of their cells. At times they even succeeded in pulling out the iron bars from the sockets of the doors.[61]

Purgatives and doses of antimony were given to the inmates of Dacca Asylum in 1841. A mixture of camphor, available at the local market, was given twice daily, both in the morning and at night, to those suffering from melancholia. It proved beneficial as a gentle stimulus. Along with this, bathing was considered an effective therapeutic component.

[59] Medical Board Proceedings, Number 7, Letter from G. Lamb to James Hutchinson, 31 October 1835.

[60] Medical Board Proceedings, Number 7, Letter from G. Lamb to James Hutchinson, 31 October 1835.

[61] Medical Board Proceedings, Letter from J. Taylor to Robert Brown, 2 May 1842.

It was believed to be the most 'efficacious means of effecting cure'.[62] According to Alexander Thomas Wise, the Superintendent of the Dacca Asylum in 1852, the treatment of mental illness in Bengal was either medical or moral, although at the same time he also agreed that some restraint was required when the patients were 'outrageous', dangerous to themselves or to others, and also when the patient refused to take food or medicine. Under such circumstances they were either confined in dark cells for hours or put on a swing. The noisy and restless patients were often put on a swing at night, because according to the superintendent, this helped to 'soothe' them and also gave them 'good sleep'. He was quite satisfied with the treatment as he found the swing to be a 'useful amusement for the most noisy and restless' patients.[63] Circulations on a swing were a form of treatment in which patients were rapidly spun around in a circular motion. The Dutch physician Herman Boerhaave (1668–1738) was the first to use such a device but the working model of a circulating swing was credited to English physician Joseph Mason Cox (1762–1822), owner of the Fishponds Asylum, Bristol.[64] As an effect of the swing, the patient often ended up vomiting, purging, bleeding from the eyes, or experienced complete disorientation followed by unconsciousness.[65] Erasmus Darwin

[62] Medical Board Proceedings, Letter from J. Taylor to Robert Brown, 2 May 1842.

[63] Alexander Thomas Wise, 'Principle Remarks on Insanity as it Occurs Among the Inhabitants of Bengal,' *Monthly Journal of Medical Science* 15 (July–December 1852), WL.

[64] For further details, see Joseph Mason Cox, *Practical Observations on Insanity; in which Some Suggestions are Offered Towards an Improved Mode of Treating Diseases of the Mind and Some Rules Proposed which it is Hoped May Lead to a More Humane and Successful Method of Cure: to which are Subjoined Remarks on Medical Jurisprudence as It Relates to Diseased Intellect* (London: R. Baldwin and T. Underwood, 1813), WL.

[65] Daniel Hack Tuke (ed.), *A Dictionary of Psychological Medicine: Giving the Definition, Etymology and Synonyms of the Terms Used in Medical Psychology With the Symptoms, Treatment, and Pathology of Insanity and the Law of Lunacy in Great Britain and Ireland*, volumes 1 and 2 (London: J. & A. Churchill, 1892), WL. Also see Richard Noll, *The Encyclopaedia of Schizophrenia and Other Psychotic Disorders*, third edition (New York: Facts on File, 1992), accessed on Google Books in November 2010.

(1731–1802), the physician grandfather of Charles Darwin also approved of the treatment for patients with different types of ailments. J. E. D. Esquirol, who called it the 'machine of Darwin', was the first to introduce it in France in 1838, although he later discouraged its use. It was also part of the regimen at Bedlam, recommended by eighteenth-century English physician John Haslam. The American psychiatrist Benjamin Rush (1746–1813), whose portrait adorns the official seal of the American Psychiatric Association, named the swing 'gyrator' or 'tranquilizer'. He approved of its therapeutic effect.[66]

Alexander Wise was not very certain about the exercise of the 'humane system of treatment' in the asylum as it required constant vigilance by the superintendents. Moreover, he stated:

> In India this cannot be relied on; and we can never calculate that the patients are not neglected, or degraded by the attendants.[67]

Instead of placing his confidence in the 'native' attendants, he found seclusion in dark rooms and the swing treatment to be appropriate measures for the effective healing of the inmates. The medical treatment included the remedy of any prominent symptoms or of certain diseases which affected the insane. Leeches were often used in local bleeding. In certain cases, the douché, or a stream of cold water, was allowed to fall from a height upon the head and neck, and cold lotions were applied. For patients whose pulse count was not strong a particular method of treatment was followed. The 'lunatic' was administered with the tartar emetic solution in doses of two or three grains every three hours, with one fourth of a grain of opium. It produced nausea and vomiting, perspiration, slow pulse rate, and a cool skin. After such agony, the patient was expected to sleep, which was also ensured by Dover's powder, which included Peruvian bark, or repeated doses of sedatives like *hen-bane* or morphia.[68] It is difficult to understand whether those were used as treatments or as punishments. The objective of the medical officer was to control the inmates and make them obey the rules, keep them

---

[66] Thomas S. Szasz, *The Manufacture of Madness, A Comparative Study of the Inquisition and the Mental Health Movement* (London: Routledge and Keegan Paul, 1971), 137–59.

[67] Wise, 'Principle Remarks on Insanity,' 111.

[68] Wise, 'Principle Remarks on Insanity,' 108.

quiet, and to get them accustomed to the asylum until they willingly engaged themselves in labour with other patients. To fulfil these aims patients had to undergo a great deal of pain. The 'hygienic treatment' of the insane in India, according to Wise, was directly related to the improvement of their general health. This was achieved in two ways: first, by employment, which involved the exercise of body and mind and second, by avoiding causes of irritation, which helped to divert the patient's attention.[69]

J. Swiney, second member of the Medical Board in 1835, believed that insanity could be cured by medical treatment. Along with medical treatment, he also adhered to 'kind treatment' and engagement in labour and other exercises for complete recovery. The remedial means implemented by him involved gentle mercurial treatment, which included blue pills (dispersed elemental mercury) along with castor oil. In instances of 'mild' symptoms of mental illness, depending on the nature of secretion, 'choylopoitic vicera' was given to the patient. J. Swiney, did not have any 'specific plan of medicine for insanity'. Therefore, in cases of irritation he yielded to bleeding and purging by blisters and by the application of 'setons' on the neck.[70]

In India, according to Swiney, the various causes of insanity were irregularities of life, distress of mind, want and deprivation of comfort and deleterious drugs which were consumed for excitement or delight; but amongst all, malaria (derived from the term, *mal aria*, or bad air) was the most important cause of mental illness. According to him, it was the most frequent and also general cause of mania, because people who suffered from fever for a long duration as well as other diseases due to malaria were prone to insanity. The primary causes of mental illness in Calcutta were the poor health conditions that predominated its suburbs, near the salt water lake in the area just outside the city, and in the jungles of Sunderbans on the outskirts.[71] Therefore, he concluded that unhealthy surroundings caused physical diseases, and prolonged illness caused by this

[69] Wise, 'Principle Remarks on Insanity,' 109.

[70] Medical Board Proceedings, Number 8, Letter from J. Swiney to James Hutchinson, 24 March 1835.

[71] Medical Board Proceedings, Number 8, Letter from J. Swiney to James Hutchinson, 24 March 1835.

finally led to insanity. This theory that ill health was caused due to tropical weather conditions and the diseases prevalent there can be well explained by the writings of James Ronald Martin[72] and W. J. Moore[73] during the early nineteenth century. According to them, Europeans of a superior constitution fell sick in the tropical climate because of its insalubrious weather conditions.

Three types of medicines were given to lunatics—purgatives, sedatives, and tonics—which were expected to control excitement and to put them to sleep. Blisters, leeches, tartar emetic solution, nitre, camphor, and occasional purgatives were given to control cerebral excitement. In 1842, A. Kean, Civil Assistant Surgeon of Moorshedabad Asylum, agreed that the effect of medicine reduced all irritation. This, along with repose and amusement or occupation, usually completed the cycle of treatment. 'Erratic maniac lunatics' were treated with an application of leeches on their necks. At times, general tonics and the decoction of bark with sulphuric acid, sulphate of quinine, and sulphate of iron were also used for their treatment. In cases of mania combined with a leprous tendency, the use of iodine was considered beneficial. In certain instances when patients refused food they were forcibly fed by stomach pumps.[74] According to the medical physicians, this led inmates to take their food voluntarily.[75] It would be hard to assume that patients would consume food voluntarily with the help of stomach pumps; rather, under such traumatic circumstances, they were actually forced to eat with the aid of such devices.

Leeches were also used for controlling maniacal paroxysms as well as to control those patients who sang and beat drums during moments of

[72] James Ronald Martin, *Influence of Tropical Climates on European Constitutions* (Calcutta: Military Orphan Press, 1841); *Notes on Medical Topography of Calcutta* (Calcutta: Military Orphan Press, 1837), NL.

[73] W. J. Moore, *A Manual of the Diseases in India* (London: John Churchill, 1861). For a detailed study, see Mark Harrison, *Climates and Constitutions: Health, Race, Environment and British Imperialism in India 1600–1850* (New York: Oxford University Press, 1999), NL.

[74] Medical Board Proceedings, Report submitted to W. Findon by A. Kean, 26 March 1842.

[75] Medical Board Proceedings, Report submitted to W. Findon by A. Kean, 26 March 1842.

'maniacal frenzy' in the Patna Lunatic Asylum.[76] This showed that although singing and drum beating was allowed in the asylum as part of moral treatment, the physicians failed to administer it properly. Hence, when inmates 'sang and drummed themselves into a state of maniacal frenzy'[77], the European officers failed to control such situations and immediately took resort to medical treatment by administering leeches on them, which they thought would both silence them and keep them under control. The Civil Surgeon at Patna, who was in favour of the medical treatment with leeches, stated that 'noisy and exciting native music, beating drums, and such like occupations were decidedly not curative means'.[78] At a time when both moral and medical treatment was practised in the asylum, the medical practitioners of asylums differed in their views. Some would practise both while others would uphold the supremacy of one method of treatment over the other. They were not really certain of the proper guidelines or the methods of administering either the moral or medical treatments as there was no defined methodology to treat mental illness. Besides, the proponents of such discussions did not distinctly express the limitations of such exercises. According to William Bynum, while the medical professionals themselves adopted many features of therapeutic programmes,

> they were not prepared to jettison their medical models of insanity, nor were they willing to compromise their central roles in the diagnosis and treatment of the mentally ill.[79]

According to A. Simpson, Superintendent of the Dacca Asylum, 'The mere physical exertion that the lunatics underwent under the morbid state of mind often exhausted them.' This frequently resulted in 'aversion to food and want of sleep'. Under such circumstances, patients were given doses of sedatives and tonic.[80] In an asylum, the reasons for

[76] Bengal Proceedings, Medical Department, Number 5, Report on the Patna Lunatic Asylum for the Year 1859.

[77] Bengal Proceedings, Medical Department, Number 5, Report on the Patna Lunatic Asylum for the Year 1859.

[78] Bengal Proceedings, Medical Department, Number 5, Report on the Patna Lunatic Asylum for the Year 1859.

[79] Bynum, 'Rationales for Therapy in British Psychiatry,' 331–2.

[80] *Annual Reports and Returns of the Insane Asylums in Bengal, for the Years 1862–66*, by J. McClelland, Officiating Principal Inspector General, Medical

inmates' physical exertion were mainly their constant engagement in asylum labour, side effects of mechanical restraints, and also general ill health from which the patients often suffered. The effect of strong dosage of medicines often led to lack of interest in food and lack of sleep.

A. Payne, Superintendent of Bengal Asylum in 1862, admitted that although medical treatment was required to cure the physical diseases of the patients, it was not effective for their mental condition. At times, blisters, setons, and other surgical means were as useless as the use of straitjackets and waistcoats.[81] Narcotics were not used, although tincture[82] of hysomus was found to be the most useful.

The asylum superintendents did not completely yield to medical treatment, while at the same time, they could not overlook its positive effects. For instance, in 1868, in the Dinajpore Asylum, the superintendent resorted to kind behaviour, healthy food, sufficient clothing, and, gradually engaging the patients in work. In addition to this a due regulation of the bowels by alternatives and aperients and the administration of tonics were given to the inmates whenever it was found necessary.[83] Bloodletting by the application of leeches was practised in asylums until the widespread introduction of medical therapy and its prescriptions of pills replaced it. For instance, bleeding and blisters were regularly used in the Moorshedabad Asylum until 1821 and were thought useful.[84]

In 1868, the Superintendent of the Patna Asylum practised bloodletting by frequently applying between three and twelve leeches to lunatics, giving narcotics to procure sleep for the restless, and tartar

---

Department, NAI. The Report on the Dacca Lunatic Asylum was submitted to W. Thomson, Deputy Inspector General of Hospitals by A. Simpson, Superintendent, Insane Hospital, Dacca.

[81] Arthur Payne, 'Annual Report on the Dullunda Lunatic Asylum, 1862,' submitted to Dr H.M. Macpherson, Secretary, Principal Inspector General, Medical Department, NAI.

[82] Tincture is an alcoholic extract of leaves, or other plant material.

[83] Home Department, Public Proceedings, The Deputy Inspector General of Hospitals to Major A. Fleming, 15 July 1868. This was sent as a reply to Sir James Clark's questions as to the cure and treatment of 'lunatics' in India, NAI.

[84] Medical Board Proceedings, Number 39, Letter from Russell to James Jameson, 25 May 1821.

emetic[85] to allay excitement.[86] At the same time, application of leeches was not in practice in the Moydapore Asylum. Instead, only 'narcotics' were used extensively in certain instances. In cases of acute mania, and in the occasional paroxysms of excitement, which was considered by the medical officers as very common among 'natives', a dosage of hypodermic of acetate of morphia (1/6 to 1/4 grain) was followed. Narcotics were given in the form of digitalis[87] in half doses of the tincture. Tincture was used when the pulse count was 'normal'. Tincture of 'hyoscyamus', in one and two 'drachm doses', was given in suitable permits. Bromide potassium was given in twenty grain doses thrice a day. Those inmates who exhibited much restlessness and sleeplessness, with absence of acute symptoms, were generally administered such dosages. In several cases, the superintendent stated that the medical treatment proved beneficial when continued for various weeks. Counter irritants, such a croton oil, tarter emetic ointment, and the liniment iodine mentioned in the *British Pharmacopoeia* (established in 1864, it is an annual publication which provides the official standard for pharmaceutical and medicinal products), were more frequently prescribed than any other drugs, especially in cases of dementia and the less acute forms of mania. Tonics and nutritious diet were generally supplied under all circumstances. According to James Wise, the constitution of the large majority of the inmates was shattered by repeated paroxysms of excitement. Physically, they were weak and exhibited a general deterioration of health due to anaemia. He further stated that among many of the inmates, proper diet along with the discipline of the asylum, the absence of all irritating causes, and the novelty of everything around them produced rapid recovery, and was found to be the best of all therapies.[88]

[85] Tartar emetic has irritant emetic properties and may cause lethal cardiac toxicity, among other adverse effects.

[86] Home Department, Public Proceedings, Memorandum from G. Saunders, 5 June 1868.

[87] Digitalis is a drug that strengthens the contraction of the heart muscle, shows the heart rate and helps eliminate fluid from body tissues. Digitalis is derived from the foxglove plant. http://www.americanheart.org (accessed on 5 April 2015).

[88] Home Department, Public Proceedings, Letter from James Wise to William Keates, 24 June 1868.

In the Dacca Lunatic Asylum, port wine with quinine, was given as a medicine to anaemic and cachetic patients. A tincture of *chiretta* was also administered. It was prepared by mixing equal parts of water and rum with chiretta. This bitter mixture was used as a stimulant tonic.[89] Although there was a tendency to include Ayurvedic medicine for treatment like chiretta, those were rare instances. This showed that the treatment of the insane in India was also based on a humoral understanding of insanity, but the treatment practised by the asylum physicians was predominantly based on European medicine.

James Wise made some interesting observations on the treatment of insanity as practised in Hindu and Unani medicine. According to Hindu medicine, he stated, the treatment of mental illness consisted of cold douches, consumption of cooling sherbets produced from coconut milk, and of a combination of carminatives with aperients. Vegetable oils, such as those obtained from the almond and violet flower, were rubbed on the scalp. The patients were often put in a dark room in their own homes. He further stated that to treat a patient, they were even 'beaten with a whip' by their family members. In some parts of the Bengal, frog soup was used as a remedy for insanity.[90] Among the *feringees*, by which he meant the 'degenerate descendants' of the Portuguese, a living frog was fastened on the top of the shaven scalp. This, according to James Wise, was considered to be a sovereign remedy for extracting the 'morbid heat', which caused mania. He also commented on the treatment of mental illness with Unani medicine. According to Unani physicians, madness originated from weakness or disorder of the humours of the brain, as well as from an excess of blood or bile. When the patient was robust, he bled. Under such circumstances, they prescribed purgatives: whey (maulijobin) with manna, twenty to thirty ingredients of electuaries, antispasmodics, and, carminatives. The asylum physicians also recognized demonic possession. To expel the devil, they used amulets on which verses of the Koran were written, charms of various kinds,

[89] *Annual Reports and Returns of the Insane Asylums in Bengal for the Years 1862–66*, J. McClelland.

[90] Home Department, Public Proceedings, Letter from James Wise to William Keates, 24 June 1868.

or burnt a piece of paper beneath the patient's nose, on which certain cabalistic words could be traced.[91]

Prophylactic medicines such as sulphate of cinchonidine, iron, and sulphuric acid were regularly and systematically given to the inmates of the Dullunda, Dacca, Patna, and Cuttack asylums with satisfactory results. The Superintendent of the Berhampore Asylum was, however, not inclined to think much of the usefulness of sulphate of cinchonidine because of his negative experiences. He recommended their usage on patients based on the report of the superintendents of other asylums. According to him, no judgement should be made on the value of a prophylactic medicine unless it was put to test.[92]

BATH: A MAJOR THERAPEUTIC FOR MADNESS

Baths were considered one of the most important therapeutics by European physicians. Medical practitioners prescribed it for 'lunatics' whenever they thought it to be necessary. Its impact was twofold. First, regular baths helped in cleansing the patient, avoiding skin diseases such as scabies, which was at one time a frequent occurrence in the asylums, and ensuring cleanliness and hygiene. Second, an occasional application of hot and cold bath was a method of treatment for mental illness, which was probably a very violent method. Bathing, like other forms of treatment, involved a direct encroachment into the private body parts of patients. Therefore, in the absence of any privacy, whether the inmates were bathed in an open space inside the asylum or outside in the river, it amused others present in the surroundings. Asylum keepers were specially appointed for bathing duties, and a 'native' doctor was placed in charge of this department. For example, in the Dacca Lunatic Asylum, both male and female patients were bathed daily. With the exception of those in hospital suffering from any particular disease, every individual was given a cold shower at least once a day. There were two shower baths

[91] Home Department, Public Proceedings, Letter from James Wise to William Keates, 24 June 1868.

[92] *Annual Report of the Lunatic Asylum for the Year 1898*, Letter sent to Colonel T. H. Hendeley, Inspector General of Civil Hospitals, Bengal from to the Secretary to the Government of Bengal, Financial and Municipal Department, dated 14 March 1899 (Calcutta: Bengal Secretariat Press, 1899), NAI.

in the asylum—one for males and the other for females. Large masonry cisterns were used to store and supply water by means of a plug, which alternately opened and closed. Water fell from a height and patients were made to stand below that for more than half a minute.

Patients who were employed in various indoor labour duties bathed inside the asylum under the shower or in a common water tank. Those employed in outdoor labour bathed in the river. On Sundays, almost all of them were taken to the river for a bath, under the supervision of an attendant.[93] It is difficult to accept that all the patients could swim. Even if it is believed, and with attendants being specially appointed to escort them, it still cannot be ascertained how safe it was to take inmates to a river in their state of mental illness. The probable reasons for this act could be that bathing in the river is a very old and widespread Indian practice, particularly for those residing in the villages. Therefore, patients were taken to the river for a bath. Second, it could also be a part of their recreation every Sunday. Third, it could have been a remedy to deal with the water scarcity in the asylum. Superintendents of asylums often mentioned such scarcities. Four, bathing was used as a means of unpaid labour, where patients not only washed their clothes but also fetched water from the river for drinking and washing. For instance, river water used for cooking and drinking was brought in a cask on a light cart by a 'water party' of eight patients under the charge of a keeper.[94] Finally, a plunge in cold water was expected to cure insanity.

The dirty and intractable patients at Dacca Asylum were particularly rubbed with *khullee* (mustard oil waste), which was made into a thin paste with water, and then washed under the shower. This 'native' substitute for soap was known to cleanse the skin and make it soft, unlike soap, which according to the superintendent, made the skin dry. Emaciated patients were rubbed daily with oil and given tepid warm water baths.[95]

---

[93] *Annual Reports and Returns of the Insane Asylums in Bengal for the Years 1862–66*, J. McClelland.

[94] Report on the Dacca Lunatic Asylum for the Year 1862, Report from A. Simpson, Superintendent, Dacca Lunatic Asylum to W. Thomson, Deputy Inspector General of Hospitals, Dacca; *Annual Reports of the Insane Asylums in Bengal for the Years 1862–66*, J. McClelland.

[95] *Annual Reports and Returns of the Insane Asylums in Bengal, for the Years 1862–66*, J. McClelland.

According to the superintendent of the asylum, baths were rarely used as a therapy at the Dacca Asylum for purposes other than that of cleanliness.[96] Those rare instances involved cold douches during high fever and shower baths in a few cases of acute and periodic mania, particularly when the patient was diagnosed with cerebral congestion. Cold bath was more frequently administered in the asylums because hot bath, according to the superintendent, was far too weakening in the tropical hot weather unlike its usage in Europe for prolonged periods.[97]

In the Patna Lunatic Asylum, other than the usual bathing routine, the cold douche was used to allay 'over-excitement' of the patient. In the Moydapore Asylum, inmates bathed daily in cold water, and water was forcefully poured over those who did not bathe voluntarily. Cold douches were administered to control those patients who suffered from 'violent excitement'. This was monitored by pouring cold water in a continuous stream of water on their back usually to cover the head and neck, from large water bags held up from a height. The medical practitioners considered this to be the most beneficial method of treatment. The process was certainly very painful, but according to the medical officer, it 'had a most salutary effect' on the patients. Unlike at the Dacca Asylum, hot bath treatment was practised in the Moydapore Asylum. It was either administered in a common tub where all the patients took their bath, or the patient was immersed in steam, enclosed inside a blanket.[98] Bath therapy was often considered a better option than the control of 'dirty' patients subdued by 'native' staff. For instance, by 1876, when dysentery was frequent in the asylums of Bengal, the superintendents could not manage 'dirty' inmates, who had the habit of putting their unclean hands into the water used for bathing or drinking. Due to this he found it difficult to eradicate dysentery from the asylums. This he thought could be relieved by putting patients under shower baths. According to him, when shower baths were introduced in the female ward of the asylum, the results were excellent. It not only helped to control dysentery,

[96] Home Department, Public Proceedings, Letter from James Wise to William Keates, 24 June 1868.

[97] Home Department, Public Proceedings, Letter from James Wise to William Keates, 24 June 1868.

[98] Home Department, Public Proceedings, Memorandum from G. Saunders, 5 June 1868.

but also helped in the overall cleansing of the patients, particularly amongst women whom the physicians considered more prone to these problems.[99]

Bath was a popular means of treatment in the West, but in India, at a time when a proper water supply system was yet to be established in asylums, bath as a means of treatment of mentally ill patients was difficult to organize. For instance, in 1872, at the Dullunda Asylum, there was no proper regular supply of water. The asylum did not have the provision of hot water baths within the asylum compounds. Therefore, patients were taken to the nearest spot outside the asylum for bath.[100] The failure of asylum managers to make such necessary provisions made patients an object of public spectacle under such circumstances. According to Surgeon R. Bird of the Dullunda Asylum, an asylum in Europe was no longer considered complete in its means to health and cure if it was not furnished with a system of douches and hot and cold baths. If this was necessary in England, it was still more essential in a hot country like India. Yet the only bath at the asylum was a shower bath in the women's yards, and it was used daily by an average of seventy-eight women. From these cases, it was evident that effective application of water for the cure of insanity and for the maintenance of health was crucial to the officials.[101] Hot plunge baths were used for the sick, mainly for those who were 'feeble and bed ridden'[102] in hospitals.

According to James Curie, physician at Liverpool and Fellow of the Royal College of Physicians at Edinburgh, Darwin established a connection between convulsive diseases and insanity, and particularly of their relation with each other. According to him, convulsive

---

[99] *Annual Report on the Insane Asylums of Bengal for the Year 1876*, by J. Fullarton Beatson, Surgeon General, Indian Medical Department sent to the Secretary to the Government of Bengal, Judicial Department (Calcutta: Bengal Secretariat Press, 1877), NAI.

[100] *Annual Report on the Insane Asylums of Bengal for the Year 1872*, by J. Campbell Brown.

[101] *Annual Report on the Insane Asylums of Bengal for the Year 1872*, by J. Campbell Brown.

[102] For further details on hot and cold baths in Hanwell Asylum in Britain, see John Conolly, *The Construction and Government of Lunatic Asylums and Hospitals for the Insane* (London: John Churchill, 1847), 40–1, WL.

diseases arise from inordinate action in the muscles and maniacal diseases arise from the inordinate action in the organs of the senses. As the muscles and the sense organs were the instruments of the will, the diseased actions both, according to him, fell under one single category, which he called 'Diseases of Volition'. The cold water treatment was considered the most effective treatment for paroxysms of both insanity and convulsions. Curie further pointed out that even in their most violent forms, the body temperature was low, and even if it increased, the heat was retained by the body with great effect.[103]

Dr Harrington Tuke, medical practitioner (1826–88) and Fellow of the Royal College of Physicians, in *On Warm and Cold Baths in the Treatment of Insanity* explained how the treatment of several forms of insanity was related to the different methods of administering baths in the asylum. Being a medical practitioner, he accepted the advantages of baths in the treatment of mental illness and also classified it into two divisions. First, baths at a temperature of or below 75° Fahrenheit included plunge bath, shower bath, and douche. Second, baths at a temperature of or above 85° Fahrenheit included hot, warm, and tepid bath. Therefore, he suggested that even if the practice was painful, it could at least be done with a controlled modulation.[104] But nowhere did the physicians in the Bengal asylums mention the temperature monitored for hot and cold baths or the method of administering it. Therefore, it is difficult to know how the treatment was administered.

OCCUPATIONAL THERAPY

According to Robert Gardiner Hill, no patients—whether male or female—should be compelled to work. Instead, they should voluntarily make themselves useful and industrious.[105] However, the application

[103] James Curie, *Medical Reports on the Effects of Water Cold and Warm, as a Remedy in Fever and Febrile Diseases, whether Applied to the Surface of the Body, or Used Internally* (Liverpool: J. M. Creery, 1804), 186–7, WL.

[104] Harrington Tuke, 'On Warm and Cold Baths in the Treatment of Insanity,' in *The Journal of Mental Science*, edited by John Charles Bucknill, Volume 45, no. VII, (1863): 532–52 (London: Association of Medical Officers of Asylums and Hospitals for the Insane).

[105] Hill, *A Concise History*, 131.

of such theories in practice was doubtful. Although Bengal asylum records show that force was not applied and labour was done by lunatics voluntarily, in reality, control always persisted. The various kinds of hard labour, which lunatics always had to perform while they were suffering from various maladies, were dreadful. It showed that some form of force was definitely applied in order to make people who were physically and mentally unwell perform such activities. Or else, one has to conclude that those admitted in the asylums were not insane, but 'sane' people who were capable of doing such laborious jobs.

In 1835, patients at the Insane Hospital of Calcutta were employed in gardening. The convalescent patients were employed in gardening, digging, weeding plants, and other 'gentle'[106] exercises. The patients were also made to whitewash the asylum, do repair work with plaster as well as construct the *machan*s on which they slept.[107] At the Dacca Lunatic Asylum too, under the Civil Surgeon G. Lamb, patients were employed in gardening and other similar activities. He complained about getting female patients to do any work in the asylum while at the same time he employed them in *soorky* or brick pounding,[108] which involved a lot of physical strength. Brick pounding work increased in the asylums with the expansion of the Public Works Department. Women did not voluntarily do the job of soorky pounding.

John Conolly had pointed out that sedentary labour was less conducive to the recovery of patients than active labour. He further stated that:

> More women get well who are employed in the kitchens, laundries, and wards than in the workrooms; and more men recover who work in the gardens and on the farms than in the tailors' or shoemakers' shop.[109]

This outlook towards a gendered division of labour was also enforced in the asylums of Bengal. James Mills had pointed out that 'the gendered

---

[106] Medical Board Proceedings, Number 8, Letter from J. Swiney to James Hutchinson, 24 March 1835.

[107] Medical Board Proceedings, Number 8, Letter from J. Swiney to James Hutchinson, 24 March 1835.

[108] Medical Board Proceedings, Number 7, Letter from G. Lamb to James Hutchinson, 31 October 1835.

[109] Conolly, *The Construction and Government of Lunatic Asylums*, 79

division of labour was intended to reinforce sex identities that the British thought proper'.[110] For instance, according to the Surgeon of the Patna Lunatic Asylum, 'women were particularly good hands at the shelling and picking of the seed'.[111]

Women in Bengal's asylums were employed more in indoor activities like spinning, weaving, and threading, while men did gardening, brick pounding, and fetching water for the asylum. But the point was that even indoor labour required a lot of strength. For instance, a lot of women were engaged in soorky pounding. According to James Wise, it was carried out in the asylum in two ways. Women were provided with a wooden lever or *dhenkee* fixed in the centre. They had to press it with their feet, which crushed the brick placed underneath the hammer fixed at its end. Men did the same job in a different way. They were provided with iron pestles to pound the bricks.[112] Both involved a strenuous process. Therefore, it was not a question of indoor or outdoor labour, and who was engaged in which; rather, it was about laborious manual labour which both were involved in and equally affected by. The asylum officials of Bengal repeatedly stated that women were employed in less strenuous jobs and were mainly engaged in indoor activities. But they chose to overlook the fact that those indoor activities also required a lot of hard work.

In 1841, patients at the Dacca Asylum were also employed in soorky pounding for the construction of roads, gardening, and heavy work like carrying water from the tank in order to wash the wards and cells. They also assisted in cooking, and repaired straw mattresses on which they slept. There was no respite from work for any of the inmates. Often they were impelled to build and maintain the asylum where they lived as patients. The physicians considered it necessary, as a part of moral

[110] James Mills, '"More Important to Civilise than Subdue"? Lunatic Asylums, Psychiatric Practice and Fantasies of "the Civilising Mission" in British India 1858–1900,' in *Colonialism as Civilising Mission: Cultural Ideology in British India*, edited by Harald Fischer Tiné and Michael Mann (London: Anthem South Asian Studies, 2004), 179–90.

[111] Simpson, 'Report on Patna Lunatic Asylum for 1871,' *Annual Report on the Insane Asylums of Bengal for the Year 1872*.

[112] Home Department, Public Proceedings, Letter from James Wise to William Keates, 24 June 1868.

treatment, to make them work. They anticipated that an involvement with labour would work as therapy. Even inactive inmates were forced to work. For instance, according to the Civil Surgeon of Dacca, those patients who were not active were put to work to make twine and mattresses and mend clothes and blankets.[113] The work assigned to the patients of the Dacca Asylum in 1843 included weeding in the garden, carrying water from the wells and tank, working in the cook room, making and repairing straw pallets, and carrying rations from the bazaar. Female patients were employed in making soorky, cleaning cotton, and spinning thread.[114] By 1852, according to the Superintendent of the asylum, Alexander Wise:

> The difficulty of finding occupation for the women was greater than for the men, as it had never been exacted from them compulsorily; and their love and habit of inactivity, prevented many from exerting themselves.[115]

There was always a general note of complaint amongst the superintendents and the medical officers of the asylum about making inmates work, irrespective of the fact that they were employed in asylum labour daily. In the Dacca Asylum, women worked for an hour before breakfast, and for about four hours after that. Every morning, some of them washed the wards, while others cleaned the cotton. Spinning, knitting, sewing, and other domestic occupations were introduced in the asylum particularly for female inmates. The superintendent claimed that he found it easier to employ men in gardening, cultivating the soil, digging, weeding, fetching bricks from the town in small carts and pounding those, or other even for heavier activities, because most of them were cultivators.[116] He probably overlooked the fact that many of the female patients admitted in the asylum were labourers or cultivators or were employed in similar jobs before being admitted.

[113] Medical Board Proceedings, Letter from J. Taylor to Robert Brown, 2 May 1842.

[114] Medical Board Proceedings, Number 18, 1843, Letter sent to Robert Brown, Superintending Surgeon, Dacca by J. Taylor, Civil Surgeon, Dacca, dated 13 April 1843, NAI.

[115] Wise, 'Principle Remarks on Insanity,' 33.

[116] Wise, 'Principle Remarks on Insanity,' 32–3.

J. Sutherland, in his annual report on the Patna Lunatic Asylum in 1859, stated that he did not 'wish to make Patna Asylum a House of Correction'.[117] His idea of treatment was of one without coercion. He was so convinced by the ideas of moral treatment of the insane that he saw to it that the labour by inmates was voluntary and the insane were 'well fed, kindly treated, and carefully attended to'.[118] He commented that patients were often unwilling to leave the asylum even after recovery. This was probably an exaggeration. It was not the kind treatment that held them back. Instead, many were not certain of their place of return and this probably made them stay back in the asylum. This was particularly so in the case of female patients.

In 1861, at the Moydapore Lunatic Asylum, inmates were employed to manufacture their own clothes and also the *morah*s, or small cane stools. Considerable profit was realized from the sale of the products manufactured by the inmates, which, according to the Superintendent Surgeon, was practised to obtain additional comforts for the patients. The profit was used to purchase blankets and new clothes for the lunatics. In certain cases, a sum of Rs 3 or Rs 4 was also given to the patients when discharged, especially to those who had no relatives or friends, so that they could sustain themselves for a few weeks after they left the hospital.[119] Similar instances were also prevalent in Moorshedabad Asylum. The profit derived from the sale of articles manufactured by the inmates, as per the order of the Secretary of State, was used to procure 'little indulgences for the patients themselves'.[120]

[117] Bengal Proceedings, Medical Department, Number 5, Report on the Patna Lunatic Asylum for the Year 1859.

[118] Bengal Proceedings, Medical Department, Number 5, Report on the Patna Lunatic Asylum for the Year 1859.

[119] General Proceedings, Medical Department, Number 4, February 1862, Report on the Moydapore Lunatic Asylum for the Year 1861, Berhampore, dated 1 January 1862, WBSA.

[120] General Proceedings, Medical Department, Number 5, 1862, Letter sent to Principal Inspector General, Medical Department from H. Bell, Officiating Junior Secretary to the Government of Bengal, dated 4 February 1862, WBSA.

Dr J. Forsyth's comment on the Patna Lunatic Asylum showed how occupation was valued as an important part of treatment. He stated that:

> Occupation, as a means of preserving and improving the general health and tranquilising the nervous system, and thereby facilitating the cure, has been attended with excellent results.[121]

In the Patna Lunatic Asylum, except for the 'idiots', a special category of inmates, a large amount of profitable work was derived from all the other patients engaged in various activities. Occupation, according to Dr Forsyth, helped to reduce paroxysms of mania among them.[122]

The inmates of the Dacca Asylum in 1862 were employed in almost every kind of indoor labour. These included rope making, soorky pounding, basket and morah making, tinsmith's work, gardening and carpentering, tailoring, *jhānp* and bamboo work, wheat grinding, domestic duties, cooking, fetching river water, keeping the grounds in order, assisting the keepers and sweepers, and attending to the sick.

The Superintendent of the asylum, A. Simpson, stated:

> As occupation was so essentially necessary in the treatment of the insane I have endeavoured as far as possible, to give them occupation without taxing their physical strength, and without using coercion, the great object being to make occupation subservient to health and not to profit.[123]

In the Patna Lunatic Asylum in 1862, John Balfour, the Deputy Inspector General of Dinapore Circle, agreed with the Superintendent as to the positive effect of making patients work. According to Balfour, not only did all curable cases improve more rapidly when the patient began to work, but the incurables also greatly benefited. Employment was considered as an outlet for the 'superfluous energy' of the violent inmates. At the same time, the poor 'imbeciles' exhibited some energy in what

---

[121] General Proceedings, Medical Department, February 1862, Annual Report of the Insane Hospital of Patna for the Year 1862 sent to E.H. Lushington, Secretary to the Government of Bengal from Dr J. Forsyth, Principal Inspector General, Medical Department, dated 18 February 1862, WBSA.

[122] General Proceedings, Medical Department, Annual Report on the Insane Hospital of Patna for the Year 1862, sent from Dr J. Forsyth to E. H. Lushington, 18 February 1862.

[123] *Annual Reports and Returns of the Insane Asylums in Bengal, for the Years 1862–66*, J. McClelland.

they undertook, and improved in health from the exercise. A large majority of the patients at the Patna Asylum were employed in work without any undue pressure being exercised. Superintendents were often eager to establish a large return from the labour of the patients. This, according to Balfour, proved his efficiency in managing the inmates in an asylum as well as his superiority to the superintendents of other asylums. Even when there was no profit, then too there was an ample return in increased and more rapid recovery among the curable patients, and in the greater quietness and happiness of the incurables. One very striking result of the effects of judicious labour was that there was no necessity for restraint.[124] Therefore, the main argument was that employment replaced restraint. But how far this was true in reality was debatable. The medical officials, after all, did not keep any statistics to prove the effect of labour on the cure of the insane.

Medical officials always emphasized the noble intentions of work without coercion as well as its healing aspects on inmates. The therapeutic ideology behind it was that if they were removed from work they would be more unruly; therefore, it would be more difficult to control them. Patients were made to operate under all circumstances because the medical officials believed that the symptoms of mental illness often subsided under industrial occupation.

The officials also pointed out that patients were not engaged in labour for any profit but for the treatment of their malady. But the profit derived from occupation was used for the benefits of inmates, for instance, for buying their goods or for paying for the establishment that looked after them. Therefore it may be argued that patients were made to do productive work, and that their work also yielded profit for the institution.

The officials of each asylum had different views about the profit of labour. For instance, unlike the official at the Patna Lunatic Asylum who pointed out that profitable work could not be derived from inmates, the Superintendent of the Dacca Lunatic Asylum employed the 'idiotic', 'imbecile', and more intractable inmates in the task of soorky pounding, earthwork, gardening, and in the oil mill for pressing mustard seeds. The profit from the labour of patients was viewed as a totality, and was not classified in the category of their diseases. Given that they were also

[124] Report of the Deputy Inspector General of Dinapore Circle, John Balfour, 1862, NAI.

employed in asylum labour, there was an attempt to extract profit from their labour as well, even though the asylum officials doubted the extent of such profit.

Every employment in the asylum was calculated. For instance, when the cost of the mustard seed in the market went up, the officials decided to stop the production of mustard oil in the asylum because they realized that the occupation was 'scarcely remunerative'.[125] In another instance, after the introduction of carpentry in the Dacca Asylum under the supervision of a carpenter hired for the hospital, the inmates manufactured almirahs, tables, and chairs, which the Superintendent stated had a 'ready sale in the city'.[126] In 1881, according to A. Payne, the Superintendent of Dacca Asylum, the amount of profit at Dacca was always higher than in any other asylums. This was because manufactured articles were sold outside the asylum at an advantageous price, instead of using them for the asylum.[127] In yet another instance, the Superintendent of the Patna Asylum discarded his initial plan of introducing a dairy farm inside the asylum due to the cheap rate at which milk was sold at the market, which would mean that the investment would not have been profitable.[128]

For deriving profit from the manufactures, inmates were even made to do additional work. For instance, a patient employed in carpentry spent five hours on such work and then spent the rest of the day in other occupations.[129] The Superintendent of Dullunda Asylum also expressed similar opinions regarding the beneficial effect of employment on the well-being and cure of the patients. He stated that the benefits of labour

[125] *Annual Reports and Returns of the Insane Asylums in Bengal, for the Years 1862–66*, by J. McClelland.

[126] A. Simpson, 'Report on the Dacca Lunatic Asylum for the Year 1862,' *Annual Reports of the Insane Asylums in Bengal for the Year 1862*, J. McClelland, Officiating Principal Inspector General, Medical Department (Calcutta: Calcutta Gazette Office, 1863), NAI.

[127] *Annual Report of the Lunatic Asylums for 1881*, by A. Payne, Surgeon General for Bengal (Calcutta: Bengal Secretariat Press, 1882), NAI.

[128] Home Department, Medical Proceedings, Number 197, June 1893, 'Report on the Lunatic Asylum of Bengal for the year 1892,' J. A. Bourdillon, Officiating Secretary to the Government of Bengal, NAI.

[129] A. Simpson, 'Report on the Dacca Lunatic Asylum for the Year 1862,' *Annual Reports on the Insane Asylums of Bengal for the Year 1862*.

and the remuneration derived from it were of secondary consideration. His aim was to make labour voluntary. According to him, the point of difference between the labour of the patients and of prisoners in jail was that while the former was expected to do labour voluntarily and not under any compulsion, the latter was expected to do the reverse.[130] But in reality voluntarily labour was hardly practised in the asylum. The kind of labour they had to engage in showed that it could not be done voluntarily. It was certainly not possible to make a physically and mentally ill person work for so many hours without using compulsion or intimidation at some level.

The primary motive of employment, according to A. Payne, was to establish a method and habit for industry, so that both profit as well as remedial and disciplinary means were achieved. The profit, according to the superintendent, would help to reduce the burden of the state for the maintenance of the Dullunda Asylum. He expressed his satisfaction over the fact that the inmates contributed towards making the institution self-supporting in a big way and labour and discipline was regulated judiciously. Patients were employed in garden labour, soorky making, gunny weaving, twine spinning, and stone breaking. Those who showed skill and aptitude were employed in more productive activities.[131] This demonstrated that they had to do more labour and thereby undergo more stress.

Coaxing was also used as a form of control. For instance, the asylum reports claimed that

> not only compulsory efforts and punishment for not working had been studiously avoided, at the same time every inducement by humouring their fancies, and granting them some coveted indulgence in diet, and extras had been employed to form a habit.[132]

[130] *Annual Reports on the Lunatics Asylums for the European and Native Insane Patients at Bhawanipore and Dullunda for 1856 and 1857,* Selections from the Records of the Government of Bengal (Calcutta: John Gray, Calcutta Gazette Office, 1858), NAI.

[131] Arthur Payne, 'Report on the Dullunda Lunatic Asylum, 1862,' sent to Dr H.M. Macpherson, Secretary, Principal Inspector General, Medical Department, NAI.

[132] *Annual Reports and Returns of the Insane Asylums in Bengal for the Years 1862–66,* by J. McClelland.

In 1879, the government ordered that a certain amount of profit from the labour should be credited to the account of the patient.[133] But according to superintendents of different asylums, inmates preferred things like tobacco, sweetmeats, and cheroots over money. For instance, at Dullunda, the practice was to reward good work with certain indulgences like these. The superintendent further stated that the sum that would accumulate as credit in favour of those inmates who would be freed after a point was too small to be useful on discharge. Moreover, as clothing and the passage home are already provided for such persons, nothing further seemed to be required. Dr Stewart of the Cuttack Asylum stated that the attempt to provide for a direct interest on the outcome of labour to the inmates was not successful. According to him, they neither cared for money nor valued it. Instead, they preferred tobacco, fruit, and other indulgences. At the Berhampore Asylum, the money so credited was spent on trifling treats and comforts. Most of the patients preferred an extra allowance of tobacco. Some spent their money on sweetmeats, others on milk and *dahi* (curd). At Dacca, money was given only to inmates of 'better intelligence'.[134] They, therefore, preferred that such work should be unpaid.

The superintendent admitted that 'compulsion in some form was necessary'.[135] Idle patients were employed with a working group with the expectation that they would be influenced by others which would make it easier for the officials to control them.

In 1870, regarding the industrial production at the Dullunda Asylum, the Surgeon A. J. Payne commented that

> the effect of work on health had been most diligently watched throughout. No consideration of profit had been allowed to prevail over the great objects of its introduction — discipline and cure.[136]

Payne tried to reduce the burden of work in the asylum by distributing heavy work, like soorky pounding or work at the oil mill, amongst

[133] *Annual Report of the Insane Asylums in Bengal, 1879*, A.J. Payne, Surgeon General for Bengal (Calcutta: Bengal Secretariat Press, 1880), NAI.

[134] *Annual Report of the Insane Asylums in Bengal, 1879*, A. J. Payne.

[135] *Annual Report of the Insane Asylums in Bengal, 1879*, A. J. Payne.

[136] K. McLeod, *Annual Report on the Lunatic Asylums, Vaccinations and Dispensaries, 1870.*

several inmates unlike other asylums. He not only reduced the hours of work but also did not impose any fixed rule for daily returns.[137] Although Payne's 'generosity' reduced the onus of work for each individual, his real intention was to make the work quicker and also increase the production.

In 1869, the Deputy Inspector of Hospitals G. Saunders visited the asylums of Bengal and commented on the kind of labour and its impact on the treatment. His observations on the European Lunatic Asylum revealed that labour was not a significant part of the asylum management there. According to him, the situation at the Bhawanipore Lunatic Asylum was different from the other 'native' lunatic asylums. Although he admitted that labour always helped to cure different forms of mental diseases, yet patients were hardly engaged in any labour. It seemed there was considerable difficulty in organizing any kind of work at the asylum just because inmates were only there for a short while. While soldiers, who constituted an important proportion of the asylum's population, hardly worked, female patients of the asylum were engaged in certain kinds of activities like needle work and crochet.[138] Dr Bird, the Superintendent of the European Asylum in 1872, stated that the task of getting inmates to work was easier at a place where they spent most of their lives, unlike in the European Lunatic Asylum where they stayed for a short period before being sent off to England.[139] This illustrated that their duration of stay functioned as a pretext for not engaging European male patients in any sort of work. But the real reason went much deeper than this. It was a matter of class. Waltraud Ernst had pointed out that the reason why employment was not an important task for the European Lunatic Asylum was that Europeans of any social class

[137] K. McLeod, *Annual Report on the Lunatic Asylums, Vaccinations and Dispensaries, 1870.*

[138] Annual Inspection Report of the Bhawanipore Asylum by G. Saunders, Deputy Inspector General of Hospitals, in *Annual Report on the Insane Asylums of Bengal, 1869*, J. Murray (Calcutta: Bengal Secretariat Office, 1870), NAI.

[139] *Annual Report on the Insane Asylums of Bengal for the Year 1872*, by J. Campbell Brown, Inspector General of Hospitals, Indian Medical Department to Secretary to the Government of Bengal, Fort William, dated 20 June 1873 (Calcutta: Calcutta Central Press Company Limited, 1873), NAI.

considered it inappropriate to debase themselves by carrying out tasks which the 'natives' could do.[140]

G. Saunders' moderate observations on labour at 'native' lunatic asylums were different from the views of superintendents and other medical officers. According to him, the objective with which 'native' asylums were established was to give shelter and medical aid to 'poor creatures'[141] who, due to their mental illness, could neither take care of themselves nor be provided for by their relatives. Therefore, it was 'most desirable that no occupation should be allotted to them'.[142] But he also stated that if at all it was necessary to engage these patients in asylum labour as a 'curative agent', the profit of the industrial fund should not be 'brought forward or exhibited as a means of lowering the expenses of attendant on the support of the institution'.[143] Moreover, he considered machine work as a better substitute for manual labour. Therefore, he introduced looms and other similar occupations at Patna Asylum,[144] which he thought were less laborious than manual work like soorky pounding or manufacturing oil. He expressed this views thus:

> In one case the labour is light and the exposure to climate is small, and consequently the expenditure of vital force is inconsiderable; in the other, all the circumstances of his daily life are against the insane.[145]

Criminal inmates were employed in work. In fact, they were considered the most productive of all the lunatics and, according to John Balfour, were free from delusions or hallucinations. It was a form of moral insanity which, according to him, affected the desires and passions only. He further stated that they committed a crime under the influence of an insane impulse and at all other times they were perfectly rational

[140] Waltraud Ernst, 'Idioms of Madness and Colonial Boundaries: The Case of the European and "Native" Mentally Ill in Early Nineteenth Century British India', *Comparative Studies in Society and History* 39, no. 1 (January 1997): 158.

[141] Annual Inspection Report of the Bhawanipore Asylum, 1869, G. Saunders.

[142] Annual Inspection Report of the Bhawanipore Asylum, 1869, G. Saunders.

[143] Annual Inspection Report of the Bhawanipore Asylum, 1869, G. Saunders.

[144] Annual Inspection Report of the Bhawanipore Asylum, 1869, G. Saunders.

[145] Memorandum by the Deputy Inspector General of Hospitals, Presidency Circle, in forwarding the Report to the Inspector General of Hospitals, Number 3385, dated 19 February 1870, in *Annual Report on the Insane Asylums in Bengal in 1869*.

and orderly.[146] Therefore, they were considered fit to do any kind of labour. This view was held by other asylum superintendents as well. For instance, in 1870 at the Patna Lunatic Asylum, most of the criminal 'lunatics' were employed in weaving cloth, tape, table covers, blankets, and spinning jute. According to the Surgeon of the asylum, B. Simpson, they turned out excellent work. The non-criminal inmates made mustard oil, bricks, and soorky, and were also employed in gardening, road making, tailoring, etc.[147]

J. Campbell Brown considered exercise and occupations to be far better alternatives than the use of restraint for controlling noisy or violent patients. He regarded the practice of mild persuasion and guidance as more efficient means of suppressing over-excitement than methods of coercion, according to him, should be set aside in all asylums conducted on humane modern principles. J. Campbell was of the opinion that too much restraint in the management of the Dullunda and Patna Asylums was bad, and he wanted to discuss this issue with the superintendents and persuade them to practise it only in very exceptional cases.[148]

At the Dullunda Asylum, in 1862, labour varied with the change of season. For instance, during the rains, stone cutting was replaced by gardening. The asylum got the contract for stone-cutting from the municipal commissioners and only strongly built male inmates were employed for the job, whereas the weaker ones were employed in spinning twine throughout the year.[149]

The occupation of the indoor patients in the Dacca Lunatic Asylum in 1868 included assisting the sweepers to clean the wards and plastering the

[146] John Balfour, 'Annual Report of the Patna Lunatic Asylum for the Year 1862,' in *Annual Reports and Returns of the Insane Asylums in Bengal, for the Year 1862*, by J. McClelland, Officiating Principal Inspector General, Medical Department (Calcutta: Calcutta Gazette Office, 1863), NAI.

[147] K. McLeod, *General Report Number 3 on the Lunatic Asylums, Vaccinations and Dispensaries, 1870*.

[148] Bengal Proceedings, Medical Department, Number 21, Letter from J. Campbell Brown to the Officiating Secretary to the Government of Bengal, 27 June 1872.

[149] *Annual Reports on the Lunatics Asylums for the European and Native Insane Patients at Bhawanipore and Dullunda for 1856 and 1857*, Government of Bengal.

walls and floors of the cells with a mixture of cow dung and mud. There were two kitchens, one for the Hindus and the other for the Muslims. Separate cooks were appointed. Although inmates assisted in both the cook rooms, their religious identity was not considered significant under these circumstances. Two of the patients were engaged in baking bread or thick wheat cakes every morning. The indoor occupations of the women included cooking and sewing. Instead of female tailors, two or three male tailors assisted female inmates in sewing cloth.[150] This shows that either assistant male tailors were easily available, or that medical officers trusted their efficiency levels more than that of female tailors. While the process of segregation in the European Asylum was based on class, in the 'native' asylums it was limited to issues of caste and religion. Therefore, discussions mainly centred on a division between Hindus and Muslims and separate arrangements were made accordingly. The position of the Superintendent of Asylums was controlled by Europeans while 'native' doctors were appointed to the posts of assistants. Indian officers, according to Waltraud Ernst, were appointed to ensure that upper-caste Hindu inmates were kept at a distance from those of the lower castes. They also made sure that Hindus were separated from Muslims.[151]

Male patients of the Dacca Asylum were engaged in the manufacture of rope and twine, and women in spinning wool. The expense of raw material like jute, or Indian flax, and wool was derived from the monthly contingency bill. To accustom the patients to regular occupation, they were both persuaded and encouraged, but under no circumstance was 'compulsion or harsh treatment' enforced. It showed that the labour of the patients, which was claimed to be perfectly free and voluntary, was somewhat deficient in 'regularity and quantity'.[152] Inmates worked in the garden, wove clothes, and blankets, and also prepared the strip of

[150] *Annual Reports on the Lunatics Asylums for the European and Native Insane Patients at Bhawanipore and Dullunda for 1856 and 1857*, Government of Bengal.

[151] Waltraud Ernst, 'Madness and Colonial Spaces—British India, c. 1800–1947,' in *Madness, Architecture and Built Environment: Psychiatric Spaces in Historical Context*, edited by Leslie Topp, James E. Moran, and Jonathan Andrews (New York: Routledge, 2007), 221.

[152] *Annual Reports on the Lunatics Asylums for the European and Native Insane Patients at Bhawanipore and Dullunda for 1856 and 1857*, Government of Bengal.

sack on which they slept at night. The women spun thread, cotton, and wool. During the summer, they were encouraged by the Superintendent to make bricks.[153] By 1871, industry constituted the principal feature of the management of Bengal asylums.[154]

In a resolution recorded in the report for 1870, the Inspector General of Hospitals, J. Campbell, was asked by the Medical Board to report whether any portion of the so-called industrial funds were 'credited to general revenues, or in any way expended on the maintenance of the lunatics'. He reported that no money realized on account of the products of inmate labour was placed to the credit of the government. Instead, it was given to the superintendents, who expended it at their discretion, and devoted it mainly for the provision of appliances for the development of industry and the purchase of raw materials. In this way, though not actually credited to the state, these funds had effected a saving of public money, because all the expenditure which was thus incurred would otherwise be defrayed by the government.[155] By 1871, the industrial system was fully implemented and the labour was turned to the full advantage of the government. It was also used for the clothing and diet of the patients. A large swamp was converted into a garden, which produced fruits and vegetables in abundance, both for consumption and for sale. Oil and soorky making, spinning and weaving, and an infinite variety of industries produced large sums of money, which was used for the improvement and the advancement of the system. According to A. Payne:

> The tanks, the large drains, the numerous expensive buildings and the good stock of machinery and appliances, were the return, which the institution was able to make to the Government for the profits of the labour hitherto surrendered by the state, which was applied to the comfort and advantage of inmates.[156]

[153] Home Department, Public Proceedings, 18 December 1868, Memorandum from G. Saunders, M. D., Deputy Inspector General of Hospitals, Lower Provinces, number 809, Dinajpore, dated 5 June 1868, NAI.

[154] Letter Number 346 from J. Campbell Brown, Inspector General of Hospitals, Indian Medical Department to the Officiating Secretary to the Government of Bengal, Fort William, dated 27 June 1872, in *Annual Report on the Insane Asylums in Bengal for the Year 1871.*

[155] Letter Number 346 from J. Campbell Brown, *Annual Report on the Insane Asylums in Bengal for the Year 1871.*

[156] A. Payne, 'Report on the Dullunda Lunatic Asylum for 1871,' *Annual Report on the Insane Asylums in Bengal for the Year 1871.*

Labour at the asylum was not considered a remedy, but instead looked upon as a source of profit. Profit from the income was used either to pay the asylum staff, or to buy these extra incentives for the inmates. The idea of work was also to make the asylum self-sustaining. For instance, rice consumed by the patients was produced within the walls of the asylums. They also wove their own clothing, beddings, and blankets.[157]

Surgeon General Hutcheson, Officiating Inspector General, reported the unsuitability of certain kinds of labour exacted from the insane in Bengal. But according to H. H. Risley, this was not communicated to the government. The Lieutenant Governor wanted a special report on the subject. Risley further stated that lunatics should not be called upon to do any penal labour. The intention was to keep them engaged, which would 'keep them from moping'.[158] According to John Conolly,

> Forcing the patients to work against their will, compelling them to work in one kind of work when they prefer another, and prohibiting the employment which they prefer; as well as the use of threats, the limitation of their diet, and recourse to devices for mortifying the patients who are indisposed to work, are faults not often … committed in asylums; but they are not unknown, and they are of a nature to be overlooked in the pride of a long list of patients employed.[159]

RECREATIONAL THERAPY

Other than engagement in various occupations, the European medical officers also allowed the 'lunatics' to engage in certain recreational activities. This, they thought, would help to cure symptoms of mental illness. In one particular instance, the Superintendent of the Dacca Lunatic Asylum took the initiative to introduce education among the patients. At a time when most of those admitted in the asylum came from the lower classes with little or no educational background, this was an ambitious project. Also, in their state of mental illness, how far such

---

[157] *Annual Report on the Insane Asylums of Bengal for the Year 1872*, by J. Campbell Brown.

[158] Home Department, Medical Branch, Number 52, September 1900, 'Annual Report on the Lunatic Asylums of India for 1899,' by E. N. Baker, Secretary to the Government of Bengal, NAI.

[159] Conolly, *The Construction and Government of Lunatic Asylums*, 80.

ideas could be implemented into practice was questionable. Besides this, the most prevalent form of entertainment included cards, games, music, or watching *nautch*es. Performances of nautches were probably meant for upper-class 'native' lunatics, although reports did not mention this, probably because it was a matter of dishonour for an upper-class 'native' to be recognized as a 'lunatic'. Yet the kind of entertainment that was provided hinted at their presence in the asylums.

EDUCATION

The asylum attendants provided instructive and amusing books written in Bengali to those patients who showed any disposition to learn. However, work was always the priority. Therefore, patients who were fit for work were not allowed to read books during working hours. Despite earlier attempts to introduce education in the Dacca Asylum, it was finally introduced in 1860. Books used in schools, and also educational prints, were purchased from the profit of their labour.[160] A. Simpson of the Dacca Asylum was enthusiastic about education in the asylum, but he finally stopped it. According to him, it was difficult to educate the 'imbeciles' as little progress could be made with them. Since the superintendents had to write reports on their duties, there was a competition amongst them to do their best and achieve something different from other asylum superintendents.

Another reason why the superintendent discontinued teaching was because he was not paid separately for this extracurricular activity. However, he continued to teach those who were disposed to learn. According to him, many of the inmates were inclined towards learning and reading the books given to them.[161] Not all the asylums adopted the same curriculum for teaching. For instance, education was not attempted in the Dullunda Asylum. According to its superintendent, the aim of the system was to restore the functions of the brain through healthy physical exercises and by

[160] General Proceedings, Medical Department, Number 11, August 1862, Letter sent to W. Thomson, Deputy Inspector General of Hospitals from A. Simpson, Superintendent of Dacca, dated 25 February 1862, WBSA.

[161] A. Simpson, 'Report on the Dacca Lunatic Asylum,' sent to W. Thomson, Deputy Inspector General of Hospitals, Dacca, in *Annual Reports of Insane Asylums of Bengal for the Years 1862–66.*

calling forth the external associations under which the brain first grows into activity in childhood. He further stated:

> Practically the simplest and most rational plan was to endeavour to revive the brain from decay by imitating the course of nature in its original growth. Habits and associations were the soil in which the ideas of childhood first sprung up, and in proportion to the care with which the former was regulated was soundness of the latter.[162]

As most of the patients admitted at Dullunda had a 'rare and scanty' record of education, it was through discipline and physical exercise that he wanted to achieve his aims. He further stated that the object of education was to restore to the brain its earlier capabilities, not to press new acquisitions upon it while it remained dysfunctional. Therefore, instead of education, the superintendent employed the 'hopeless idiots' in manual work of the asylum, as he considered them capable of performing such physical tasks better. The patients received rewards according to their diligence. In private asylums, which already had some educated inmates, were found to take to study as an easy and healthy exercise. However, according to the superintendent, these cases were rare in the pauper asylums of India, particularly in Bengal.[163]

The Superintendent of the Moydapore Lunatic Asylum also tried to introduce education. *Darogas* (constables) were placed in charge of this duty. The patients were divided into three different classes, depending on the type of their insanity. Those who showed good progress received tobacco or sweetmeats as incentives.[164]

GAMES AND AMUSEMENTS

The medical officers wanted to strike a balance between work and leisure. Therefore, patients were also engaged in various kinds of games as a part of their recreational therapy. Patients frequently amused themselves with games that involved light physical exertions.[165] In 1852, while acting

[162] A. Payne, *Annual Report on Dullunda Lunatic Asylum, 1862.*

[163] A. Payne, *Annual Report on Dullunda Lunatic Asylum, 1862.*

[164] Superintendent J. M. Coates, 'Report on the Moydapore Lunatic Asylum for the Year 1872,' *Annual Report on the Insane Asylums of Bengal for the Year 1872.*

[165] Medical Board Proceedings, Report submitted to W. Findon by A. Kean, 26 March 1842.

as the Superintendent of the Dacca Asylum, A. Wise involved them in various kinds of amusements and recreational activities. They were made to sit on the verandas or on the grass and amuse themselves. According to him, their favourite amusement consisted of *panchese*, which was a kind of draughts and cards. This was usually played by 'natives' with a small amount of money, but inside the asylums, they were not allowed to play the game with money. Another source of amusement was music. They often played on the hand drum, also known as *tom tom*. Animals such as deer, sheep, and cows were brought into the asylum for their amusement. Patients took interest in feeding and attending to them, which the superintendent thought 'awakened and exercised the social and benevolent feelings'.[166] The different forms of entertainment introduced by Dr Strong at Dullunda Asylum included singing, dancing, card games (not gambling), and 'native' musical instruments.[167]

Inmates were allowed to play games or musical instruments only after their evening meal. 'Tractable' and 'well-behaved' lunatics were occasionally allowed to go out to the bazaar, with attendants, particularly during the festivals. They even went outside the asylum to sell the manufactured goods.[168] As the selling of manufactured goods involved financial transactions, such an act raises questions about the real nature of their mental illness.

A group of inmates sang and made 'discordant' sounds with the 'native' guitar and cymbals. They enjoyed the noise thoroughly and joined in the chorus. Monthly nautches were held, which only the 'better behaved' and 'industrious' lunatics were allowed to attend. Inmates enjoyed such performances. No impropriety was permitted, and any noise or interference with the singers or players was punished by the immediate removal of the patients from that place. However, according to the medical officers, such a practice was seldom necessary.[169]

[166] Wise, 'Principle Remarks on Insanity,' 34.

[167] *Annual Reports on the Lunatics Asylums for the European and Native Insane Patients at Bhawanipore and Dullunda for 1856 and 1857,* Government of Bengal.

[168] A. Simpson, 'Report on the Dacca Lunatic Asylum,' sent to W. Thomson, Deputy Inspector General of Hospitals in *Annual Reports and Returns of the Insane Asylums in Bengal for the Years 1862–66.*

[169] Home Department, Public Proceedings, Letter from James Wise to William Keates, 24 June 1868.

Amusements became so much an established and recognized part of the treatment of the insane that according to the superintendent, it became necessary to conduct it in a 'regular and systematic manner'.[170] According to G. Saunders,[171] the manners and customs of the natives of Bengal were entirely at variance with those in England. Therefore, the different kinds of amusement of the former were also much different from the latter. The amusements were briefly described as follows: a 'native' would, at a certain period of the year, go wild after kite flying. He sat for hours and listened with rapture to the monotonous beat of a drum, the horrid drone of the national pipe, or the squall of the dancing girl. If he had any spare copper or cowries, he gambled with them, or gorged himself at a sweetmeat shop and stupefied himself with palm juice, or maddened his brain with *ganja*. Therefore, the inmate was helpless when he was left to himself. His knowledge of reading and writing was only sufficient to enable him to look after his rupees, *anna*s, and *pice*. Even if he could read more, there was no literature available, and due to the 'uncouth' written characters, he failed to read what he had written. Therefore, when insanity clouded such a mind, there was not much to lose, and a very little went a long way in amusing the afflicted mind. He had his kite to fly, his drum to beat, and he played cards with his fellow inmates. In return, he was given a bit of tobacco leaf. If he could win wrestling matches, he received a cigar from the superintendent as a prize. Patients took their daily walks outside the walls, or spent an hour on the merry-go-round. The Superintendent of the Patna Lunatic Asylum allowed the poor patients unlimited latitude and to the best effect.[172]

Therefore, a 'therapeutic rationale' was constructed within the asylum to achieve short-term objectives. The emphasis on moral treatment changed the discourse on the inmates and the way insanity was observed and understood. It replaced the old horror tales of the asylum as a place of severe torture and physical coercion, and helped to look at the asylum as a place where the humane treatment of mentally ill persons took place with care and patience. 'Restraint was the grand substitute for inspection,

---

[170] Scull, *The Most Solitary of Afflictions*, 285.

[171] Home Department, Public Proceedings, Memorandum from G. Saunders, 5 June 1868.

[172] Home Department, Public Proceedings, Memorandum from G. Saunders, 5 June 1868.

superintendence, cleanliness and every kind attention.'[173] The treatment of 'lunatics' varied over time as well as differed from one asylum to the other. The asylum reports by the superintendents throughout the nineteenth century stated that the patients were provided with all types of benefits and cures inside the asylum. The implementation of labour without the use of any kind of force was considered a successful way of treating inmates. Manual labour meant great physical exhaustion and the result was expected to produce a relatively docile and manageable inmate. How far insanity could be cured by engaging them in various forms of labour voluntarily or involuntarily is questionable.

The medical supervisors attempted to implement what they considered to be the best possible method of treatment in the respective asylums. In the process of doing so, they yielded to all forms of treatment—medical, mechanical, and moral. Over time, the combination of moral and medical treatment helped the definition of insanity to take shape, as it was otherwise impossible without knowing how and what form of treatment was applied for its cure. By the end of the nineteenth century, the much recognized procedure of moral treatment gradually lost its significance. Insanity began to be known as a medically curable mental disease. This established the supremacy of medical therapy over the moral therapy. Moral treatment even in its humane form proved to be extremely harsh. But medical treatment along with its prescriptions of dosages was equally or even more bitter.

[173] Conolly, *The Construction and Government of Lunatic Asylums*, 28.

3

WOMEN IN THE LUNATIC ASYLUMS OF BENGAL

THIS CHAPTER LOOKS AT WOMEN diagnosed as insane and the treatment that followed to cure them in the European and 'native' asylums of Bengal in the nineteenth century. It studies the social background of the women admitted to the asylums and attempts to classify the different causes and symptoms of mental illness among them. Definitions of insanity always remained fluid. It seemed more difficult to define 'mad women' than 'mad men' in the asylums. The causes of mental illness among the former remained mostly 'unknown' at the time of their admissions. This category included those cases where the causes of insanity were not known. For instance, out of forty-one female patients admitted at the Dullunda Asylum in 1862, the source of the maladies for thirty cases were 'unknown' (see Table 3.1). There were many such instances and the table only cites one such instance.

Therefore, in case of 'unknown' patients, 'descriptive rolls' could not be maintained. Although this category consisted of both men and women, it can be concluded from the annual reports of asylums that there were more women than men who fell in this category. At a time when the definition of insanity itself was in the making and the medical practitioners were trying to understand the differences between male and female insanity, the category of the 'unknown'

Table 3.1 Annual Returns of 'Native' Female Insane Patients Treated in the Asylum at Dullunda during the Year 1862, Showing 'Unknown' Cases

Names	Age	Occupation	Caste	Birth place	Diseases	Cause	Cause of death
Omourto	63	Unknown	H	Bengal	Mania Chronic	Unknown	
Belatone	42	,,	M	,,	,,	,,	Asthenia
Murtoo	33	,,	H	,,	,,	,,	
Jeerah	42	,,	M	,,	Monomania	,,	
Sallee	40	,,	CH	,,	Mania Acute	,,	
Manee	50	,,	,,	,,	Dementia	,,	
Dooknee or Peerun	32	,,	M	,,	Mania Chronic	,,	
Petteme, prisoner	43	,,	H	,,	,,	,,	Dysentery
Unknown, Boba	32	,,	,,	,,	,,	,,	
Kameenee or Rajee	26	,,	,,	,,	,,	,,	
Purressmonee	38	,,	,,	,,	,,	,,	Asthenia
Taree Kouranee	26	,,	,,	,,	,,	,,	
Jeebnee or Jhannobee	35	,,	,,	,,	,,	,,	
Sonah	50	,,	M	,,	,,	,,	Asthenia
Cowsullah	27	,,	H	,,	,,	,,	
Armon	43	,,	M	,,	,,	,,	Dysentery
Pecohree	50	,,	H	,,	,,	,,	
Dookee	25	,,	,,	,,	,,	,,	
Deenoe or Joymonee	40	,,	,,	,,	,,	,,	

(Cont'd)

Table 3.1 (*Cont'd*)

Names	Age	Occupation	Caste	Birth place	Diseases	Cause	Cause of death
Topsee	15	,,	CH	,,	,,	,,	
Doorgee	23	,,	H	,,	,,	,,	
Unknown, Surfee	33	,,	,,	,,	,,	,,	
Monglah, prisoner	25	,,	,,	,,	,,	,,	
Rushnee	27	,,	M	,,	Mania Acute	,,	
Talleeoh	30	,,	H	,,	Mania Chronic	,,	
Rossmonee	25	,,	M	,,	Mania Acute	,,	
Mulleeka	50	,,	H	,,	Mania Chronic	,,	
Hosainee	30	,,	M	,,	Mania Acute	,,	
Norkish	22	,,	CH	,,	Imbecility	,,	
Neemee	35	Juggee	H	,,	Dementia	,,	
Unknown, Number 39	35	Unknown	,,	,,	Melancholia	,,	Dysentery
Ahnah	30	,,	M	,,,,	Mania Acute	,,	Dysentery
Sumputee	60	,,	,,	,,	Melancholia	,,	Asthenia
Unknown, Number 44	40	,,	,,	,,	Dementia	,,	
Ullungo	28	,,	H	,,	Mania Acute	,,	Asthenia
Rammonee	35	,,	,,	,,	,,	,,	Dysentery
Surjee	30	,,	,,	,,	Imbecility	,,	
Beemolah or Beemoh	18	,,	M	,,	Mania Acute	,,	
Beendoo	40	,,	H	,,	,,	,,	
Asseemum	35	,,	M	,,	Mania Chronic	,,	

Name	Age		Diagnosis	Cause	Outcome
Gholabee	18	H	Mania Acute	,,	Diarrhoea
Unknown, Soorjee, Number 47	28	,,	Melancholia	,,	,,
Luchmonee	34	M	Mania Acute	,,	Diarrhoea
Mohorum	30	,,	Mania Chronic	Ganja Smg.	Asthenia
Tarramonee	30	H	Mania Acute	Unknown	
Showba	30	,,	,,	,,	
Buckee, Unknown, Number 48	35	,,	Mania Chronic	,,	
Bissasee	10	CH	Amentia	Congenital	
Obhoyoh	40	M	Mania Acute	Unknown	
Kissorree	30	H	,,	,,	
Settah Raur	30	,,	,,	Ganja Smg.	
Assoorun	50	M	,,	,,	Dysentery
Parbutty	35	H	,,	,,	
Alladee	25	,,	,,	Unknown	
Mungaun	50	M	,,	,,	Asthenia
Rannee	38	H	Mania Chronic	Ganja Smg.	
Saddee	30	,,	Mania Acute	Unknown	
Rannee	38	,,	Mania Chronic	Ganja Smg.	Dysentery
Rushnee, alias Sugnee	30	,,	Mania Acute	Unknown	

Source: 'Annual Returns of 'Native' Female Insane Patients Treated in the Asylum at Dullunda during the Year 1862' in *Annual Reports and Returns of the Insane Asylums in Bengal*, compiled by J. McClelland (Calcutta: Military Orphan Press, 1863), NAI.

further complicated the situation. It was not possible to know about the prior history of the illnesses of many women admitted into the asylums. The insane were usually admitted in the asylums by their friends, relatives, and acquaintances, and this helped the medical officers to maintain a prior case history of the patients along with their 'descriptive rolls'. It was a record-holding book, which included a detailed chronicle of the patients, for instance their name, age, place of birth, cause of illness, date of admission and release. The treatment began with recording the case history on the patient's admission. The availability of prior history made it easier for the physicians to address patients' illnesses. Initial symptoms of the illness were noted in prior case histories, which were usually narrated to the physician by the family members who first observed any difference in the nature or characteristics of the patient, unless the patient had already visited a local physician. Family members, therefore, helped the physicians to understand the patient's physical or mental problems. The physicians often expressed their discontent over the unavailability of prior case histories and they often criticized the 'natives' as ignorant. This was because the physicians were not specially trained to treat mental patients.

The spatial segregation of women in the European Lunatic Asylum was not based on mental disorders, but rather on their class composition which was divided into three categories: upper, middle, and pauper classes. They were usually supported by their friends, relatives, or acquaintances, unlike in the 'native' asylums where inmates were by and large maintained at the expense of the government until the late 1870s, when the government introduced a fixed monthly payment to be paid at the time of admission. Case studies of women in the European Lunatic Asylum showed how difficult financial situations often caused their transfer from rooms to wards maintained at public cost. Upon admission to the asylum, European women had to get accustomed to their place of confinement. Moreover, a modification of lifestyle due to the transfer of status from upper class to lower class worsened their situation. Therefore, European women faced several problems after admission in the asylums in addition to their physical and mental illnesses which had already weakened them.

A. Fleming, the Official Civil Surgeon of the Moorshedabad Lunatic Asylum, stated in 1862 that 'institutionalised lunatics' mostly belonged to the poorer classes of the community.[1] He further stated that women—other than those who wandered on the streets as friendless *faqueer*s (wanderers), the bazaar girls, and criminals—were usually not sent into the asylum at Moorshedabad. This conclusion was based on his understanding of the 'manners and habits' of local people. According to the medical officers, all the inmates of the asylums in Bengal, whether men or women, belonged to the lower sections of the society. This class of people mainly comprised prostitutes, vagrants, and beggars, as well as cultivators' wives, barber's wives, female cultivators, fisherwomen, and so on. These details were available from the records of descriptive rolls, which the medical officers could fill in on certain rare occasions, during the time of admission.

By 1871, statistics showed that the majority of the patients admitted belonged to the lowest and least educated classes.[2] Amongst the patients of the Moydapore Asylum, by 1872, the male population mainly consisted of cultivators whereas beggars made up the female population.[3] The social composition of women continued to be the same until 1875, when, in Dullunda, there were two beggars, five coolies, one fisherwoman, one housewife, eight prostitutes, three domestic servants, one washerwoman, and twenty-two 'unknown' cases among female inmates. At Dacca there were two *grihisti* or housewives, one domestic servant, one beggar woman, and one 'unknown' case. Amongst the women admitted at Patna, there were three cultivators, one beggar, one labourer, one prostitute, one domestic servant, one shopkeeper, one weaver, and one from another occupation, in addition to five 'unknown' cases. At Cuttack in the same year, an insane woman worked as a coolie before she was admitted to the asylum. At Berhampore, there were four cultivators, one labourer, two domestic servants, and one from some

---

[1] A. Fleming, 'Report on the Moorshedabad Lunatic Asylum for the Year 1862,' NAI.

[2] *Annual Report on Insane Asylums of Bengal for the Year 1871*, by J. Campbell Brown, Inspector General of Hospitals, Indian Medical Department (Calcutta: Bengal Secretariat Press, 1872), NAI.

[3] Superintendent J. M. Coates, 'Report on the Moydapore Lunatic Asylum for the Year 1872,' *Annual Report on the Insane Asylums of Bengal for the Year 1872*, by J. Campbell Brown, Inspector General of Hospitals, Indian Medical Department to Secretary to the Government of Bengal, Fort William, dated 20 June 1873 (Calcutta: Calcutta Central Press Company Limited, 1873), NAI.

other occupation.[4] At Dullunda, in 1885, there were two beggars, one maid servant, one potter, one prostitute, and one teacher. Eight women were not involved in any sort of occupation, and one female patient had no prior history. At Dacca there were seven cultivators, one beggar, and one Christian missionary. At the Patna Asylum, there were five beggars, two cultivators, two labourers, and two undertakers, while Berhampore admitted one beggar, one cultivator, and three female patients whose case histories were not known.[5]

Medical officers faced difficulties in knowing the exact details of an inmate's age and previous history of illness. This, according to them, was not only the situation for those patients who were picked up from the streets by the police and admitted into the asylum, but also for those who were admitted by their family, friends, or by other acquaintances. According to James Wise, a wandering 'lunatic' picked up by the police could hardly give any account of himself or herself. At the same time relatives were so 'ignorant and unobservant of dates' that exact details were impossible to procure. The absence of prior case histories resulted in the medical officers criticizing the 'natives' as 'ignorant and uneducated'.[6]

Of the total number of Europeans and East Indians treated at the European Lunatic Asylum, eighty were men and twenty-one were women. Amongst the East Indians, ten were men and thirteen were women. Amongst the Europeans, however, sixty-four were men and only eight were women. This difference, according to the superintendent, was because the number of European men in India was much greater than the number of European women.[7] This was true because

[4] *Annual Report on the Insane Asylums of Bengal for the Year 1876*, by J. Fullarton Beatson, Surgeon General, Indian Medical Department (Calcutta: Bengal Secretariat Press, 1877), NAI.

[5] Home Department, Medical Board Proceedings, Number 131, July 1886, Letter number 137 sent to R. H. Wilson, Officiating Secretary to the Government of Bengal from A. J. Cowie, Inspector General of Civil Hospitals Bengal, dated 4 June 1886, NAI.

[6] James Wise, 'Report on the Dacca Lunatic Asylum for 1871,' in *Annual Report on Insane Asylums of Bengal for the Year 1871.*

[7] R. Bird, 'Report on the Bhawanipore Lunatic Asylum,' *Annual Report on the Insane Asylums of Bengal for the Year 1872.*

most of the European patients admitted there were soldiers. Hence, by drawing a comparison between numbers of men and women, the superintendent tried to point out that although fewer women were admitted, insanity was in no way a rare occurrence amongst the European women settled in India.

The proportion of female patients admitted in the asylums of England was always higher than men. For instance, the data collected in England and Wales by the Royal Commissioners in Lunacy suggested that institutionalized women outnumbered men in 1880 by about 7,000. The total number of women was 39,027 and that of men was 32,164.[8] This was not the situation in India, and particularly not in Bengal. For instance, in 1865, out of fifty-six Hindu patients, forty-seven were male and only nine were female; amongst fifty-eight Muslims, there were fifty-one males and seven females.[9] According to Waltraud Ernst,

> the phenomenon that women are more likely than men to be diagnosed as mentally unstable has become part of feminist orthodox in the West.[10]

In 1862, the Superintending Surgeon at Moorshedabad, after judging the reports of the asylums in England, concluded that women there were just as much, or even more subject to this malady than men. According to him, this increase in the proportion of female 'lunatics' in England had no correlation with the admission of women in the asylums of Bengal.[11] Elaine Showalter in her book, *The Female Malady*,[12]

[8] R. Bird, 'Report on the Bhawanipore Lunatic Asylum,' *Annual Report on the Insane Asylums of Bengal for the Year 1872.*

[9] G. Saunders, 'Report on the Dacca Lunatic Asylum for the Year 1865,' in *Annual Report on the Insane Hospitals of Bengal for the Year 1865*, compiled by W. A. Green, Officiating Principle Inspector General (Calcutta: Military Orphan Press, 1866), NAI.

[10] Waltraud Ernst, 'Feminising Madness - Feminising the Orient: Madness, Gender and Colonialism in British India 1860–1940,' in *Exploring Gender Equations: Colonial and Post Colonial India*, edited by Biswamoy Pati and Shakti Kak (New Delhi: Nehru Memorial Museum and Library, 2005).

[11] A. Fleming, 'Report on the Moorshedabad Lunatic Asylum for the Year 1862,' *Annual Report and Returns of Insane Asylums in Bengal for the year 1863* (Calcutta: Military Orphan Press, 1863), NAI.

[12] Elaine Showalter, *The Female Malady: Women, Madness and English Culture, 1830–1980* (London: Virago Press, 1987).

pointed out that in England, insanity was more 'popular' than it was in India and, 'alongside the English malady, nineteenth century psychiatry described a female malady'. She further explained that 'even when both men and women had similar symptoms of mental disorder, psychiatry differentiated between an English malady, associated with the intellectual and economic pressures on highly civilized men, and a female malady, associated with the sexuality and essential nature of women'.[13] During the time when the understanding of insanity and its practices in the colonies was very similar to what was happening in England or in Wales, this seemed a little perplexing. In India, and particularly in Bengal, not only was the term 'female malady' unfit to define the 'madness' of women, it was also difficult to draw a conclusion on the issue as the number of women admitted to asylums in India was lower, for various reasons, than what it was in England.

In Bengal, mental illness was common among both men and women. In the mental hospitals of England and Europe, proper records with case studies were maintained of the number of women admitted to the asylums. Women were not sent into the asylum because insanity was considered as a social stigma; this was so not only in Bengal, but also the case in India in general. Women admitted to the asylums existed only as numbers in the statistical records with hardly any references to their case studies, except in a few rare instances. Therefore, it cannot be concluded that insanity was a specifically female malady. Reports revealed that insanity was a common occurrence irrespective of the gender of the patient. The complexity of the problem lay in the definition and understanding of the term 'insanity'. It was also difficult to ignore the fact that a gendered definition of mental illness was gradually taking shape where a woman's insanity was explained more in terms of the condition of her emotional state, which was at times described as melancholic and distressed while at other times as violent and outrageous. The official understanding of her insanity was often related to her emotional exuberances, for instance, her ways of laughing, singing, or talking to herself. The medical officers assumed that women in general had no control over their emotions, which often caused mental illness. Women were considered as emotionally vulnerable, and therefore, prone to insanity.

[13] Showalter, *The Female Malady*, 7.

Moore pointed out that many female European residents in India suffered from 'uterine disease' due to 'climatorial influences'.[14] This happened because 'young females', during their voyage to India from England, often got emotional upon leaving their homeland. This was followed by 'excitement consequent on a succession of new scenes', and sea sickness, and added to all these were symptoms of premenstrual cycle that worsened the situation.[15] He further stated:

> There is frequently exposure to chilling winds and moisture, neglect of suitable clothing, the tedium and fatigue of a long march up country, and, lastly, the early marriages so constantly negotiated, all powerful agents to disturb the uterine, nervous, and vascular system.[16]

Therefore, an unstable emotional condition, sea sickness, and adapting to a different climatic condition often delayed their menstrual cycles.[17] He stated that early marriages, before the 'thorough development' of the sexual organs, often led to diseases of the womb among native women. This illustrated that European physicians considered the onset and even or uneven flow of menses as a significant reason associated with mental illness among women. The lack of medical writing and discussions on women's mental health in the nineteenth century by the medical practitioners of India made it impossible to know their opinion on the association of menstrual cycle with female insanity. Moore pointed out that 'the influence of tropical climates on the rise and progress of uterine disease does not appear to have received that attention, which the subject demands from Indian medical authors'.[18] Thus the reasons for women's mental illnesses in India and in the West were understood on a similar note, thereby challenging prevailing notions of racial differences. In the absence of medical literature in nineteenth-century India on the 'uterine diseases' of women, this was not conceived as a correlated or significant explanation for women's mental illnesses.

Of the known causes, consumption of *ganja*, epilepsy, puerperal fever, and hereditary causes, were categorized as physical causes, whereas grief

---

[14] W. J. Moore, *A Manual of the Diseases of India* (London: John Churchill, 1861).

[15] Moore, *A Manual of the Diseases of India*, 129.

[16] Moore, *A Manual of the Diseases of India*, 130.

[17] Moore, *A Manual of the Diseases of India*, 130. The term 'catamenia' or 'catamenial' flow was used in medical records to define menstrual cycle of women.

[18] Moore, *A Manual of the Diseases of India*, 130.

or domestic problems were classified as moral ones. Anger, passion, melancholia, acute mania, and intemperance were classified as emotional causes of female insanity. In 1835, in a report on the Insane Hospital of Dinajpore, J. Marshall, the Superintending Surgeon, expressed his doubts about reaching any accurate conclusion regarding the comparative frequency of insanity between men and women; according to him, the 'middle life period of women was most obnoxious to insanity'.[19] He was of the opinion that puerperal[20] mania was common in India. According to medical reports, women usually faced this problem after a laborious and difficult childbirth. There were very few references to puerperal mania in the asylums of Bengal. According to the medical officers, it was more frequent among women in the European asylums than among women of the 'native' asylums. James Reid was of the opinion that

> the term puerperal insanity is not only understood to imply aberration of the mind, or derangement of the cerebral functions in the puerperal state itself, but to include those attacks which occurs sometimes during the period of gestation, as well as those which we more frequently meet with few months some months after parturition, whilst the patient is suckling her infant.[21]

According to Thomas A. Wise, Surgeon of the Dacca Lunatic Asylum, 'The variety of mental derangement incident to women soon after parturition seems to be less common in Bengal than in Europe.'[22] According to the Superintending Surgeon, as no 'decent' family permitted their

[19] Medical Board Proceedings, Number 8, 24 March 1835, Enclosure to a letter sent to James Hutchinson, Secretary to the Medical Board from Mr. Swiney, Second Member Medical Board also Superintendent Surgeon, Presidency, dated 24 March 1835, NAI.

[20] Puerperal—origin: Latin, *puerpera*; a lying-in woman; 'puer' means 'child' and 'parere' means 'to bear'. Puerperal fever is a postpartum sepsis (the presence of organisms in blood) with a rise in fever after the first twenty-four hours following the delivery of a child, but before the eleventh postpartum day.

[21] James Reid, 'On the Symptoms, Causes and Treatment of Puerperal Insanity,' reprinted from *Journal of Psychological Medicine and Mental Pathology*, volumes 1 and 2, edited by Forbes Winslow, in *Asylum Journal 2*, edited by John Charles Bucknill (1855–6), WL.

[22] Alexander Thomas Wise, 'Principle Remarks on Insanity as It Occurs among the Inhabitants of Bengal,' *Monthly Journal of Medical Science*, 15 (July–December 1852), WL.

women to be confined in a public asylum, he was frequently requested by the local people of Dinajpore to treat their female relatives at home. This hinted at the occurrence of puerperal fever outside the asylum as well. The superintendent found it difficult to judge the extent of such cases in Bengal, because within the asylum, it was not frequent, and he did not treat enough cases outside the asylum to reach a definite conclusion. According to Yannick Ripa, women with puerperal fever or mania either suffered from 'intense depression or acute frenzy'.[23] Elaine Showalter, while pointing out the frequent occurrences of puerperal insanity in England, stated that 'it seemed to violate all of Victorian culture's most deeply cherished ideals of feminine propriety and maternal love'.[24]

In Bengal, the issue of puerperal mania did not limit itself to the question of maintaining or breaking the norms of femininity. Rather, it pointed to a more complicated medical issue. It raised certain questions about the treatment of female illnesses, for instance, what led to so many cases of puerperal mania or fever? Was it related to hygiene? Did women give birth in unhygienic conditions? Therefore, this particular cause of woman's insanity questioned the status of reproductive and mental health of women as well. While much was done about women's reproductive health through the Dufferin Fund, towards the end of the nineteenth century, the issue of women's mental health was never taken into consideration by the medical officers.

The superintendents of the asylums constantly made comparisons and came to the conclusion that the number of women in the asylums in Bengal was always lower than that of the men. In 1835, at the Insane Hospital of Calcutta, the average age of males at the time they were admitted to the asylums was twenty-five years while that of women was twenty years. The number of women as compared to men was 1 to 3 or 4. Based on these records on the ratio of the sexes, the Superintendent Surgeon stated that in reality, mental illness was more frequent amongst men than amongst women in the country.[25] Even four decades later the

[23] Yannick Ripa, *Women and Madness: The Incarceration of Women in Nineteenth Century France*, translated by Catherine du Peloux Menage (Cambridge: Polity Press, 1990).

[24] Showalter, *The Female Malady*, 58.

[25] Medical Board Proceeding, Number 8, 26 March 1835, Enclosure to Letter sent from Mr Swiney to James Hutchinson, 24 March 1835.

condition was almost similar; women constituted 21.5 per cent of the admissions in the asylums of Bengal by 1871, against 23.6 per cent in 1870 and 20.8 per cent in the preceding five years. A large proportion of the admissions consisted of Hindu women, rather than Muslims: they comprised 23.76 per cent and 13.97 per cent respectively.[26]

The Inspector General of Hospitals stated that in the asylums in England, the population of insane women generally exceeded the number of insane men, whereas in Bengal, the number of women admitted in the asylums constituted only 22 per cent of the total number of patients. The number of female patients treated in the hospitals (not mental hospitals) and dispensaries of Bengal, excluding the medical institutions of Calcutta, comprised 26 per cent of the population. As the number of women treated for their mental illness outside the asylums was higher than of those in the asylum, he presumed that

> whatever the relative amount of male and female population of Bengal, or the relative number of lunatics among males and females, the people are more loath to send females to asylums, and contrive to manage them at home.[27]

According to J. Campbell, the Inspector General of Hospitals, the 'custom of the country [India] was opposed to sending women either to hospitals or asylums'.[28]

The number of women admitted to the Moorshedabad Asylum in 1842 was not above 1/6 or 1/7 of the male numbers, while in Europe the former predominated.[29] Mental illness due to consumption of substances like liquor or hemp was categorized as a moral cause of insanity. In Europe, more men were subject to this cause of mental illness than women. At Dacca, in 1835, the ratio of males to females was 4 to 1

[26] *Annual Report on Insane Asylums of Bengal for the Year 1871*, J. Campbell Brown.

[27] *Annual Report on Insane Asylums of Bengal for the Year 1871*, J. Campbell Brown.

[28] Resolution, Judicial Department, Medical, Calcutta, A. Mackenzie, Officiating Secretary to the Government of Bengal, dated 4 October 1872, in *Annual Report on Insane Asylums of Bengal for the Year 1871*.

[29] Medical Board Proceedings, May 1842, Letter sent to G. Bushby, Secretary to the Government of India from A. Kean, Civil Assistant Surgeon, Moorshedabad, dated 12 November 1841, NAI.

respectively. This, according to the superintendent, led to an uncertain indication of the relative frequency of insanity between the sexes. Certain circumstances made this deduction 'doubtful'. He condemned the 'habits' of the 'natives', which he thought was responsible for this difference. He believed that mental illness was as common among women as it was among men. By stating that all women admitted to the asylum during the year were prostitutes, he insisted that it was mostly women who were found wandering on the streets that were admitted to the asylums by the police. He claimed that to save the honour of families, 'deranged' women were often locked at home.[30]

Recoveries among male patients amounted to 22.8 per cent of the average strength for the year, and among women it was 28.2 per cent. The ratio of recoveries per cent of the admissions of the year were 47.1 and 60.4 for men and women, respectively. The experience of asylums in other countries was thus affirmed in Bengal, namely that insanity was a more curable disease among females than among males. Therefore, according to James Hutchinson, 'it would be an interesting subject of study to investigate and weigh' the difference.[31] In 1872, female inmates constituted 18.9 per cent of the total admissions in all the asylums in Bengal against 21.5 per cent in 1871 and 23.6 per cent in 1870. This showed a decrease over time. Female Muslim patients were fewer in number than both Muslim males and Hindu patients of both sexes. The number of female Christian patients was even lower. Most of the women admitted in the asylums during this period were in their 40s. According to the Inspector General of Hospitals, the proportion of female 'lunatics' was higher in the earlier decades of the nineteenth century than it was in the 1870s.[32] According to Surgeon B. Simpson of the Patna Lunatic Asylum, very few 'natives' of the lower class, especially women, were aware of their accurate age.[33] By 1872, the percentage of recovery was

[30] Medical Board Proceedings, Number 7, 9 October 1835, Letter sent to James Hutchinson, Secretary to Medical Board from G. Lamb, Civil Surgeon, Dacca, dated 31 October 1835, NAI.

[31] Annual Report on Insane Asylums of Bengal for the Year 1871, J. Campbell Brown.

[32] Annual Report on the Insane Asylums of Bengal for the Year 1872, by J. Campbell Brown.

[33] Annual Report on the Insane Asylums of Bengal for the Year 1872, by J. Campbell Brown.

greater among women than among men at the Moydapore Asylum. According to the Superintendent of Moydapore Asylum,

> their quieter lives and pettier anxieties in their family duties, their minor exposure and less hard labour, with their fewer and less injurious dissipations, left them less liable to insanity, and more easily returnable to their normal condition.[34]

Superintendent James Wise of Dacca Asylum stated that before making any comparison between the mortality rates in different asylums, it was necessary to know the class, age, previous history, and duration of patients' mental illness. Certain factors determined the death of an inmate in the asylum, which, according to him, included the distance they travelled, the mode of conveyance they used, the food given to them en route, and the physical state in which they arrived. He further stated that boats or steamers were usually used for commuting in eastern Bengal. The patients were sent from one district to another using these modes of conveyance and constables were placed in charge of those patients during the journey. When they were about to start from the zillah station, they were examined by the Civil Surgeon, who testified to their fitness for travel. Often, weeks lapsed from the date of this examination till they finally arrived at the asylum. For instance, in 1870, it took some patients twenty-eight days to arrive at Dacca Asylum from Assam, and thirteen days for others from Cooch Behar. During the journey, the principal food item was *chura* (parched rice), which was worm-eaten, or new rice, and *khisari dal* (pulses). Constables were criticized by the medical officers for not taking proper care of the 'demented' or 'refractory lunatics'. Due to the delay in initiating the journey along with long-distance travel and poor consumption of 'low grade food', patients often suffered from general debility, or from disease of the lungs or bowels, on arrival.[35]

By 1866, according to Superintendent A. Payne of the Dullunda Asylum, 'lunatics' were sent to the asylum from the surrounding districts of Moorshedabad, Bograh, Rungpore, and Rajshahye, and twenty

---

[34] Superintendent J. M. Coates, 'Report on the Moydapore Lunatic Asylum for the Year 1872,' *Annual Report on the Insane Asylums of Bengal for the Year 1872.*

[35] James Wise, 'Report on the Dacca Lunatic Asylum for 1871,' *Annual Report on Insane Asylums of Bengal for the Year 1871.*

cases were received by transfer from the Moydapore Asylum on its abolition. On learning that it was the intention of the government that the Dullunda Asylum was to receive patients from these long distances in the future, he drew their attention to the risk to life that accompanied the patients who had travelled so far. From his previous experiences on the mortality of the patients, he stated that

> it is true that the cases that have proved fatal after a long journey were all of them more or less enfeebled physically as well as mentally before the journey; but such cases must always form a portion of the lunatics of a large Civil Division and a sufficient portion to forbid, on grounds of humanity, the denial of them of an asylum within reasonable distance from their homes.[36]

He was also concerned about the hardship imposed on the patients when, after recovery, they were compelled to travel from Calcutta to Moorshedabad. Therefore, a feeble and rheumatic old woman, who was received from Moydapore, was not discharged even when she recovered her reason. She subsequently died in the asylum.[37]

The cause of insanity among both men and women, according to the Superintendent of Moorshedabad Asylum in 1842, was physical.

> That was when one or more of the mental powers or manifestations were abysmal owing to the derangement either organic or functional of the cerebral centre on which that manifestation depend.[38]

A similar view about the physical causes of mental illness was also held in 1842 by the Superintendent of the Dacca Lunatic Asylum. The physical causes, in order of their frequency of occurrence at the asylum were consumption of ganja and opium, epilepsy, intemperance, and heredity.[39] The superintendent assumed that since women were less addicted to

[36] A. Payne, 'Report on the Dullunda Asylum,' sent to H. M. Macpherson, Secretary Principle Inspector General, Medical Department, Fort William, Dullunda, dated 8 February 1866, in *Annual Report on the Insane Asylums of Bengal for the Year 1865*, W. A. Green.

[37] A. Payne, 'Report on the Dullunda Asylum,' *Annual Report on the Insane Asylums of Bengal for the Year 1865*.

[38] Medical Board Proceedings, May 1842, Annual Reports on the Insane Hospital in Moorshedabad, dated 26 March 1842, NAI.

[39] Medical Board Proceedings, Annual Reports on the Insane Hospital in Moorshedabad, 26 March 1842.

ganja-smoking than men, their numbers were fewer. He also emphasized that in India, almost 'no females excepting such as belong to the lower classes would generally be allowed to visit a public hospital'.[40]

The medical officers had repeatedly expressed their discontent over the fact that it was exceedingly difficult to obtain correct information of the causes of mental illness among those admitted in the asylums because 'lunatics' were seldom accompanied by anyone who had any knowledge of the matter.[41] This was true for both men and women. But throughout the nineteenth century, in various medical reports, the medical officers asserted the fact that this situation was more frequent with women.

Superintendent A. Payne stated that it was tougher to assign the causes of insanity amongst asylum inmates in India than in England, since in India, he noticed a reluctance among the patients to speak of their 'hereditary tendency' and to disclose the habits that had preceded the onset of the problem. Therefore, he concluded that an error might arise from mistaking those practices as causes of mental illness which were actually its first manifestations.[42]

The Superintendent of the Patna Lunatic Asylum stated that female patients admitted to the asylum suffered from chronic symptoms which often resulted in dementia. He also considered physical illnesses as the cause of insanity. But what he found problematic was the increasing physical illnesses over time, which often resulted in mental disease. According to him, 'organic disease was often present, and they were less curable as regards their mental condition'.[43] Therefore, they were more liable to fall victims to ordinary disease than cases of acute mania. Justifying the need to send in patients at an initial stage, the superintendent further stated that the mental diseases, like other diseases, were expected to be cured with comparative ease if diagnosed on time, failing which

[40] Medical Board Proceedings, Letter from A. Kean to G. Bushby, 12 November 1841.

[41] Medical Board Proceedings, Annual Reports on the Insane Hospital in Moorshedabad, 26 March 1842.

[42] *Annual Report on the Insane Asylums in Bengal, 1879*, by A. J. Payne, Surgeon General for Bengal (Calcutta: Bengal Secretariat Press, 1880), NAI.

[43] John Balfour, 'Annual Report of the Patna Lunatic Asylum for the Year 1862,' in *Annual Reports and Returns of the Insane Asylums in Bengal for the Year 1862* by J. McClelland, Officiating Principal Inspector General, Medical Department (Calcutta: Calcutta Gazette Office, 1863), NAI.

there would be a great increase in the number of permanently insane persons throughout the province.[44] Therefore, by the nineteenth century, patients were admitted at an early stage not only because their family members wanted them to be cured while the disease was in its early stages, but also because they feared that a late admission might further complicate the situation and delay the treatment.

The causes of mental illness were determined by the medical officers from the prior case studies of inmates and from their class composition, which included the 'peculiar habits, customs and feelings of the "natives" of the country'.[45] The cases admitted at the Dacca Asylum were, for the most part, either those of acute mania, when the patients were violent or dangerous, or cases of long-standing chronic mania bordering on dementia, and of dementia itself. The 'natives', according to the medical officers of the asylums, were very reluctant to send their relatives to a asylum, for anything else other than the cases of acute mania. The Superintendent of the Dacca Asylum stated that they seldom received patients for treatment during the early stages of their diseases, when it was easier for them to treat such cases successfully. The superintendent resented the fact that it was only when insanity showed itself in its violent forms and the patient was uncontrollable, or when the disease was so far advanced that the person was no longer able to share the work of the household, or had become incapable of taking care of himself or herself, that his relatives sent him or her to the asylum.[46] This complicated the situation and delayed the treatment. The intention of the medical officers was to treat maximum number of cases admitted in the asylums and to release them. But such instances not only deferred treatment, it often led to an increase in the asylum population.

[44] John Balfour, 'Annual Report of the Patna Lunatic Asylum for the Year 1862,' *Annual Reports and Returns of the Insane Asylums in Bengal for the Year 1862.*

[45] H. C. Cutcliffe, 'Report on the Dacca Lunatic Asylum for the Year 1870,' in *Report on the Lunatic Asylums, Vaccinations, and Dispensaries in the Bengal Presidency for the Year 1870*, compiled by Assistant Surgeon K. McLeod, Officiating Secretary to the Inspector General of Hospitals, Indian Medical Department (Calcutta: Bengal Secretariat Press, 1872), NAI.

[46] H. C. Cutcliffe, 'Report on the Dacca Lunatic Asylum for the Year 1870,' *Report on the Lunatic Asylums, Vaccinations, and Dispensaries in the Bengal Presidency for the Year 1870.*

According to the superintendent, the 'natives' perceived asylums as a place in which troublesome or helpless 'lunatics' were taken care of, rather than as an institution in which the disorders of the intellect may, to some extent, be successfully treated as well.[47]

By 1865, the causes of mental illness among female inmates at the Dacca Asylum remained largely 'unknown' other than a few instances of anger, passion, grief, loss of property, epilepsy, ganja consumption, and hereditary and congenital tendencies. The diseases from which they suffered were mainly chronic mania and dementia. Therefore, it could be concluded that they were either discharged as cured or absorbed back in the category of asylum staff. Reasons for complications among the remaining patients were syphilis (in two cases), paralysis (in one case), and 'cachexia' (for the remaining cases).[48] According to Superintendent James Wise, 'cachexia' depicted a general deterioration of the system. Combined with other diseases, an inmate became prone to it in the asylum. The recovery of 'cachexia' became uncertain. Therefore, the practice was to record the most prominent disease on admission into hospital and enter it in the monthly register. During the course of the illness, the patient could be affected by other diseases and the one under which the patient was admitted was often not the one he died of (see Table 3.2).[49]

Another disease that often caused the death of female patients was known as 'asthenia'. Superintendent A. Payne explained this as being the condition wherein an inmate died of physical exhaustion without assignable organic cause and unattended by marked anaemia or other evidence of blood disorder. He further stated that it expressed

only a state of slow general innutrition due to impairment of cerebral function, as the final general exhaustion of Bright's diseases, phthisis, and much other chronic affection would be rightly termed the asthenia of those

[47] H. C. Cutcliffe, 'Report on the Dacca Lunatic Asylum for the Year 1870,' *Report on the Lunatic Asylums, Vaccinations, and Dispensaries in the Bengal Presidency for the Year 1870*.

[48] W. B. Beatson, 'Report on the Dacca Lunatic Asylum for the Year 1865,' sent to G. Saunders, *Annual Report on the Insane Hospitals of Bengal for the Year 1865*.

[49] James Wise, 'Report on the Dacca Lunatic Asylum for 1871,' *Annual Report on Insane Asylums of Bengal for the Year 1871*.

Table 3.2 Annual Returns of Patients Treated in the Dacca Asylum during the Year 1865, Showing Complications in Female Inmates Caused Due to 'Cachexia'

Name	Age	Occupation	Religion or Caste	Parentage	Birthplace, Village, Pergunnah and Zillah	Diseases	Cause	Complications
Unknown Soorjeemoney	46	Ayah	C	Bengalee	Zil. Dacca	Dementia	Angry Passion	Cachexia
	40	Barber's Wife	H	Bengalee	,,	Moral Insanity	*Ganja*	Paralysis agitans
Endromoney	40	Prostitute	H	,,	,,	Mania Chronic	,,	Syphilis Secondary
Nundoo	51	Cultivator's Wife	H	,,	,,	,,	Unknown	None
Unknown (right ear split by ring)	39	Unknown	H	Asamese	Zil. Kamroop	Dementia	,,	,,
Kistomoney	41	Cultivator's Wife	H	Bengalee	Vil. Noggadah, Th. Toowargunge Zil. Chittagong	Mania Chronic	Unknown	None
Soshee Brahmunee	31	,,	,,	,,	Vil. Gourboat, Pergh. Jamala, Zil. Gowalparrah	Mania Chronic	,,	Syphilis Secondary
Goolaabee	33	,,	M	,,	Vil. Shalloar, P ergh. Servile, Zil. Tipperah	,,	,,	Epilepsy

(*Cont'd*)

Table 3.2 (*Cont'd*)

Name	Age	Occupation	Religion or Caste	Parentage	Birthplace, Village, Pergunnah and Zillah	Diseases	Cause	Complications
Shonv	32	Servant	M	,,	Vil. Esapoorah, Pergh. Toraub, Zil. Tipperah	,,	Epilepsy	None
Rajcoomaree	23	Cultivator's Wife	H	,,	Vil. Bahmeeburiah, Pergh. Shutterkindul, Zil. Tipperah	,,	Unknown	,,
Bunno	27	Unknown	M	,,	Zil. Dacca	Dementia	,,	,,
Oprakas Lame	45	Unknown	M	,,	Zil. Chittagong	Dementia		,,
Koylas	26	Prostitute	M	,,	Vil. Gopaulgunge, Pergh. Mymensingh, Zil. Mymensingh	Dementia	*Ganja*	,,
Neeksjaun	15	Cultivator's Wife	M	,,	Vil. Bohimpore, Pergh. Meharcoor, Zil. Tipperah	Dementia	Unknown	,,
Tapee	20	Domestic	H	,,	Vil. Bareeput, Pergh. Moolagool, Zil. Sylhet	Mania Chronic	,,	,,
Anunco	40	Cultivator's Wife	M	,,	Vil. Soonakandah, Th. Nursingdhee, Zil. Dacca	,,	,,	,,

Name	Age	Occupation	Sex	Race	Residence	Form of Insanity	Cause	Complications
Daggee 'alias' Bahma	40	Domestic	H	Bengalee	Vil. Furreedabad, Zil. Dacca	Mania Chronic	Unknown	None
Luckee	45	Cooly's Wife	H	"	Vil. Ghatall, Ph. Ghatall, Zil. Hooghly	"	*Ganja*	"
Maun Bee	69	Domestic	M	"	Zil. Dacca	"	Loss of Property	Cachexia (old age)
Sumput	28	Poddar's Wife	H	"	Vil. Amlegoola, Th. Laulbaugh, Zil. Dacca	"	Hereditary	None
Autter Bee	37	Domestic	M	"	Zil. Dacca	"	Unknown	"
Manick Bee	36	"	M	"	Vil. Jaun Bazaar, Th. Naraingunge, Zil. Dacca	"	"	"
Moolookjaun	16	Cultivator's Wife	M	"	Vil. Ratcoola, Ph. Bresalejur, Zil. Tipperah	"	"	Cachexia
Motee Bee	25	"	M	"	Vil. Ecuriah, Th. Paschundee, Zil. Dacca	Dementia	Hereditary	None
Phallanee	46	Domestic	H	"	Vil. Batparrah, Th. Roopgunge, Zil. Dacca	Mania Chronic	*Ganja*	"

(*Cont'd*)

Table 3.2 (*Cont'd*)

Name	Age	Occupation	Religion or Caste	Parentage	Birthplace, Village, Pergunnah and Zillah	Diseases	Cause	Complications
Noorjaun	25	Unknown	M	,,	Vil. Shobul, Th. Hatazaree, Zil. Chittagong	Mania Chronic	Unknown	None
Churdee	35	Prostitute	H	,,	Vil. Roopakhole, Ph. Alapsingh, Zil. Mymensingh	,,	Intemperance	,,
Khutzeer Bee	25	Unknown	M	,,	Vil. Nowanugger, Ph. Allapsing, Zil. Mymensingh	Dementia	Unknown	,,
Bunnoo	55	Domestic	M	,,	Zil. Dacca	Mania Chronic	Grief	Cachexia
Ayna Bee	35	Zamindar	M	,,	Mouzah Taknee, Pergh. Boraye, Zil. Sylhet	Mania Chronic	Unknown	None
Rammunnee	30	Unknown	H	,,	Vil. Patchal, Th. Sabar, Zil. Dacca	,,	Grief	,,
Tarra	50	Beggar	H	,,	Zil. Dacca	Dementia	Unknown	,,
Luckee	35	Domestic	H	,,	,,	,,	Congenital	,,
Aradhunnee	40	Carpenter's Wife	H	,,	Zil. Dacca	Mania Chronic	Hereditary	,,

Name	Age	Occupation			Residence	Diagnosis	Cause	Result
Unnoo	28	Prostitute	H		Zil. Midnapore	"	*Ganja*	Cachexia
Soomee	26	Prostitute	M	"	Zil. Calcutta	Mania Chronic	*Ganja*	"
Mullick Bewah	50	Beggar	M	"	Vil. Noya Barree Tuppa Paukhowal, Zil. Mymensingh	"	"	"
Jebun Bewah	40	Husbandry	M	"	Vil. Kamalpoor, Pergh. Soosuny, Zil. Mymensingh	Mania Chronic	*Ganja*	None
Ruzun Bewah	60	Beggar	H	"	Zil. Mymensingh	"	"	"
Comulle	56	Beggar	H	"	Zil. Dacca	Dementia	Unknown	None
Khuttejan	35	Unknown	M	"	Zil. Dacca	Mania Chronic	Unknown	"
Kaleetarah	29	Cooly's Wife	H	"	Zil. Dacca	Mania Chronic	*Ganja.*	"
Tarramoney	45	Shopkeeper's Wife	H	"	"	"	Unknown	Cachexia
Ansoe	35	Cultivator's Wife	M	"	Vil. Kaprowla, Th. Laulbaugh, Zil. Dacca	"	*Ganja*	None
Poorushee	38	Prostitute	H	"	Vil. Poorhutee, Th. Suburchur, Zil. Furredpore	Mania Chronic	*Ganja*	None

(*Cont'd*)

Table 3.2 (*Cont'd*)

Name	Age	Occupation	Religion or Caste	Parentage	Birthplace, Village, Pergunnah and Zillah	Diseases	Cause	Complications
Shalca Bewah	55	Cultivator's Wife	M	,,	Vil. Alipur, Ph. Nazirpur, Zil. Backergunge	Mania Chronic	Unknown	Cachexia (Old Age)
Abeer Bee	30	Domestic	M	Bengalee	Zil. Dacca	Mania Chronic	Unknown	None
Peertenee	35	Cultivator's Wife	H	Bengalee	,,	,,	,,	Cachexia
Jeetnee	38	Domestic	M	,,	,,	,,	*Ganja*	None
Kooshum Bee	30	Cultivator's Wife	M	,,	Mh. Hazrej, Ph. Khilta, Zil. Sylhet	,,	Unknown	Cachexia
Soonamoney	35	Unknown	H	,,	Zil. Dacca	,,	,,	None
Chundra	45	,,	H	,,	,,	,,	Unknown	,,
Noorjan	25	Domestic	M	,,	Zil. Dacca	,,	*Ganja*	None
Neckjaun	18	,,	M	,,	Vil. Gagra, Ph. Runbhowal, Zil. Mymensingh	Mania Chronic	Unknown	None
Bassar Bee	35	Unknown	M	Bengalee	Zil. Dacca	Dementia	Unknown	None

Source: Annual Report on the Insane Asylums in Bengal for the Year 1865, compiled by W. A. Green, Officiating Principal Inspector General, Medical Department (Calcutta: Military Orphan Press, 1866), NAI.

diseases, and distinguished from specific causes of death immediately arising out of the visceral disease present. The term 'exhaustion of mania', on the other hand, is applied to cases where the suspension of function is directly fatal, and finds its parallel in the uroemic convulsion of Bright's disease, the fatal syncope of a fatty heart.[50]

The report of the number of women admitted at the Dullunda Asylum in 1865 showed the number of women who died due to 'asthenia' (see Table 3.3).

By 1871, according to James Wise, melancholia was very common among 'native' patients. He further stated that men were more subject to this than women. Religious melancholia was not found among Bengalis, except among those 'natives' who had been converted to Christianity. Religious exaltation was not uncommon. It was generally characterized by great self-complacency and vanity. The individual affirmed that he was holier and more favoured by the deity than other men: that he could call down the judgement of God on the human race, or that he saw his patron god at night and communed with him.[51]

For many of the male inmates at the Dacca Asylum in 1835, insanity was found to originate in dissipation, especially in the habitual and excessive use of intoxicating liquors and drugs. It frequently happened that a man was discharged after being perfectly sane for several months and was returned in a state of raging insanity three or four days later due to the consumption of *bhang* or ganja.[52]

The onset of insanity due to the consumption of intoxicating substances, particularly ganja, was contested by medical professionals throughout the nineteenth century. Until the establishment of the Indian Hemp Drug Commission in 1893, the medical officers were in doubt about the relationship between ganja and insanity. An interesting conundrum about ganja consumption, which the medical officers could not solve, was whether it was reasonable to suppose

[50] James Wise, 'Report on the Dacca Lunatic Asylum for 1871,' *Annual Report on Insane Asylums of Bengal for the Year 1871.*

[51] James Wise, 'Report on the Dacca Lunatic Asylum for 1871,' *Annual Report on Insane Asylums of Bengal for the Year 1871.*

[52] Medical Board Proceedings, Number 7, Letter from G. Lamb to James Hutchinson, 31 October 1835.

Table 3.3 Report on Women Admitted at the Dullunda Asylum in 1865 Showing Female Inmates Who Died Due to 'Asthenia'

Name	Age	Occupation	Caste	Birth place	Disease	Cause	Cause of death
Omourtoo	64	Housewife	H	Bengal	Mania Chronic	Unknown	–
Belatone	44	,,	M	,,	,,	,,	–
Rajee or Kameenee	28	,,	H		Mania Chronic	Unknown	–
Marree	52	,,	CH		Dementia	,,	–
Jeerah	46	,,	M		Monomania	,,	Febrinous Clot in Heart (Febrinous Clot)
Unknown Bobah	34	,,	H		Mania Chronic	,,	–
Kowswalla	30	,,	,,		Melancholia	,,	Liver Abscess
Pecohree	37	,,	,,		Mania Acute	,,	–
Doorgee	25	,,	,,		,,	,,	–
Surphee	26	,,	M		Imbecility	,,	–
Tellecoh Kaloarnee	32	,,	H		Mania Acute	,,	–
Rashmonee	27	,,	M		,,	,,	–
Norkish	37	,,	CH		Imbecility	,,	–
Name Unknown	42	,,	H		Dementia	,,	–
Number 45							
Reshmee or Doorgee	32	,,			Mania Acute	Ganja Smoking	–
Bidda Goohleenee	38	,,			Mania Chronic	,,	Asthenia

Name	Age		Residence			
Surjee Raur	34	„		Mania Acute	Unknown	—
Alladee	32	„		„	„	—
Nundee	26	„		Mania Chronic	Ganja Smoking	—
Mary Drummond	26	CH		„	Unknown	—
Elizabeth Blyth	26	„		„	„	—
Hurrou	26	H		Imbecility	Epilepsy	Diarrhoea
Doorga Raur	30	„		Mania Acute	Ganja Smoking	—
Radhamonee	33	„		„	Unknown	Diarrhoea
Champa	29	„		„	„	Asthenia
Sunnechury	21	„		„	Epilepsy	—
Asseemun	36	M		„	Unknown	—
Neemee	37	H		Dementia	„	—
Poynah Bibee	61	M		„	„	—
Sreemuttee	51	H		Mania Acute	„	—
Darmoney, Prisoner	39	M	Zillah 24 Pergunnahs	„	„	Dysentery
Goolchee Bewah	51	H	Calcutta	„	„	Diarrhoea
Cammeenee	22	„	„	„	„	—
Assorun alias Archee	51	M	Zillah Jessore	Dementia	„	—
Khattoon	36	„	Zillah 24 Pergunnahs	Mania Epilepsy	Epilepsy	Dysentery

(Cont'd)

Table 3.3 (Contd)

Name	Age	Occupation	Caste	Birth place	Disease	Cause	Cause of death
Harrannee	21	„	H	Calcutta	Mania Acute	Ganja Smoking	–
Nestereenee	30	„	„	Zillah 24 Pergunnahs	„	Unknown	–
Obhoyoh	35	„	„	Calcutta	„	„	–
Essoree Number 65	40	„	„	„	Mania Chronic	„	Diarrhoea
Sreenuttee	30	„	„	„	Mania Acute	„	–
Khamah	20	„	„	„	„	Ganja Smoking	Asthenia
Raibutty	45	„	„	„	„	Unknown	–
Nusseebun	20	„	M	„	„	Ganja Smoking	–
Shodamonee	35	„	CH	„	„	Unknown	Asthenia
Parbuty	36	„	H	„	„	Ganja Smoking	–
Baichun	30	„	M	„	„	Unknown	–
Bamchund	25	„	H	„	„	Ganja Epilepsy	Debility
Gowree Dassee	26	„	„	„	Mania Puerperal	Unknown	–
Takoor Doyal	50	„	„	„	Mania Acute	Ganja Smoking	–

Name	Age		Place		Cause	
Annund Raur	28	„	Zillah Moydapore	Dementia	„	–
Gowree	55	„	„	„	Unknown	Asthenia
Soorodhunnee	37	„	„	Mania Chronic	„	Hepatic Disease Lardaceous
Chelleoh	33	„	„	Mania Acute	„	Dysentery
Sunneechurry	35	„	Zillah Howrah	„	„	Anaemia
Chundermonee	40	„	Zillah Kristonogur	„	„	–
Telloo Bewa	35	M	Zillah Moorshedabad	„	„	–
Munnajaun	45	„	Calcutta	„	„	–
Bibee Autour	35	„	Zillah 24 Pergunnahs	„	„	–
Unnow Raur	25	H	Zillah Howrah	„	„	–
Name Unknown no. 75	60	„	Zillah Jessore	„	„	Asthenia
Soorjoomonee	40	„	„	„	„	Debility
Rajissoree	22	„	Calcutta	„	„	–
Heerah Raur	17	M	„	„	Ganja Smoking.	–
Mooktokassee	25	H	„	„	„	–
Heeroo	30	„	„	Mania Chronic	Unknown	–
Surroop Raur	40	„	„	Mania Acute	„	–
Deegamburry	45	H	Zillah Howrah	Mania Chronic	Unknown	–

(Cont'd)

Table 3.3 (*Cont'd*)

Name	Age	Occupation	Caste	Birth place	Disease	Cause	Cause of death
Deeroo	25	,,	,,	Calcutta	Mania Acute	,,	–
Bhotun	35	,,	,,	,,	,,	,,	–
Samah	25	,,	,,	,,	,,	,,	–
Bamah	20	,,	CH	,,	,,	,,	–
Marian Manual	20	,,	CH	,,	Mania Chronic	,,	–
Poornoo	32	,,	H	Zillah Beerbhoom	Mania Acute	,,	–
Badshau Bibee	25	,,	M	Zillah Moydapore	Observation	,,	–
Kamenie	30	,,	H	Calcutta	Mania Acute	,,	–
Tyluck, Prisoner	22	,,	,,	Zillah Howrah	Observation	,,	–
Taramonee	55	,,	,,	,,	Mania Chronic	,,	–
Puddeo	45	,,	,,	Calcutta	Mania Acute	,,	–

Source: Annual Report on the Insane Asylums in Bengal for the year 1865, compiled by W. A. Green, Officiating Principal Inspector General, Medical Deparment (Calcutta: Military Orphan Press, 1866), NAI.

that excessive ganja-smoking caused mental illness, or whether it was the other way round.[53]

Although the European medical officers mentioned certain cases of insanity among that was caused due to the consumption of intoxicating substances like bhang, ganja or *charas* (a narcotic resin), some of them also argued that the consumption of intoxicating substances was not the real cause of insanity. In 1886, A. J. Cowie, Inspector General of Civil Hospitals, Bengal, in his annual report on the insane asylums, stated that women 'did not acquire the *bhang, ganja*, or *charas* habits and for *obvious* [italics mine] reasons'.[54] Instead, he pointed out that the majority of the cases of intoxication that were admitted to the asylum included young and middle-aged men. He stated that it was a social taboo for a woman to consume such substances. This was an attempt to guard the notion of a righteous woman who would not indulge in such activities. They tried to refer to the norms of feminine behaviour by putting forth such ideas. At a time when women's insanity was not much talked about and not many women were admitted to asylums, the possibility of female consumption of such substances complicated the issue. It broke the pattern of visualizing women as an epitome of moral values, derived from notions of the ideal upper-class Victorian woman.

Drs J. Wise and J. Coates, the two Superintendents of Dacca and Moydapore Asylums, respectively, during 1872, stated that Indian hemp was in many cases erroneously credited with 'madness'. They further stated that this drug had little or no influence as an incentive for crime. The proportion of ganja consumption resulting in mental illness among criminals, was lower among non-criminal patients. Dr Wise stated that thieves and murderers smoked hemp in order to nerve themselves for criminal deeds. But the drug was not especially capable of arousing any homicidal or criminal propensities.[55] In 1884, in the report on the

---

[53] J. A. Bourdillon, 'Report on the Lunatic Asylums of Bengal for the Year 1892,' Home Department, Medical Proceedings, Number 195, June 1893, NAI.

[54] Home, Medical B, Numbers 130–1, July 1886, Report on the Lunatic Asylums Bengal, 1885, NAI.

[55] *Annual Report on the Insane Asylums of Bengal for the Year 1872*, J. Campbell Brown.

'lunatic asylums' of Bengal, the causes of insanity were mainly attributed to the use of ganja and spirits. In this connection the Inspector General made the following remarks:

> One woman is set down as having suffered from the effects of bhang (Dullunda), while opium is alleged to have caused mental disease in another (Patna). Yet opium is said to be extensively consumed by both sexes in some districts. Spirits as a cause of insanity is largely represented. No mention, notwithstanding this, is made of 'alcoholism' or 'delirium tremens' in any of the returns.[56]

The Inspector General of Hospitals became critical of the Superintendents' views on intoxication as a cause of insanity, and therefore doubted the correctness of assigning several cases of insanity to excessive drinking. The end of the nineteenth century was the beginning of the time when medical officers began to disapprove of a possible correlation between the consumption of hemp and the cause of insanity, which they earlier agreed upon. This led him to conclude that the Superintendents' views were mere 'guess work'.[57]

The method of classifying different forms of insanity underwent revision during the year, with the objective of securing some uniformity of classification. But, as pointed out by the Inspector General, it was impossible to expect absolute accuracy and uniformity, since the diagnosis depended almost entirely on the views held by individual superintendents: while some of them considered the consumption of ganja as a fertile cause of mental illness, others thought it a rather innocuous kind of stimulant.[58] Writing about ganja smokers or other inebriates, A. Payne stated that 'their resort to a stimulant was an effect and not a genuine cause of mental failure'.[59]

It seemed that whenever a 'lunatic' was reported by the police to be a ganja smoker, it was easily assumed that the drug was the cause of

[56] Home Department, Medical Board Proceedings, Number 100, September 1885, 'Report on the Lunatic Asylums of Bengal for the Year 1884,' NAI.

[57] Home Department, Medical Board Proceedings, Number 100, September 1885, 'Report on the Lunatic Asylums of Bengal for the Year 1884'.

[58] Home, Medical, Number 10, January 1892, 'Report on the Lunatic Asylums of Bengal,' by H. H. Risley, Officiating Secretary to the Government of Bengal, NAI.

[59] A. Payne, *Annual Report on the Lunatic Asylums of Bengal for 1879.*

his or her insanity. Consumption of ganja was considered by the medical officers as one of the important causes of insanity. The Lieutenant
Governor agreed with Dr Harvey, the Inspector General of Hospitals,
that many cases from the previous years were attributed to ganja on the
most insufficient grounds. Therefore, by 1894, the whole question of
the effect of the consumption of this drug upon the social and moral
condition of the people was put under the consideration of the Hemp
Drugs Commission. Dr Harvey was convinced that their report would
undoubtedly show the extent to which the use of hemp drugs was the
cause of mental illness.[60]

In 1872, according to the Inspector General of Hospitals, the
proportion of acute insanity was lower among females than among
males. The ratio of recovery and improvement was much higher in
acute cases rather than in the chronic cases of insanity. The death
rate was highest for patients with acute dementia, which resulted
from melancholia, acute mania, chronic dementia, and chronic
mania. Alexander Wise made some observations on the phases of
mental illness. According to him, mental depression culminating in
suicide was very common among both Muslims and Hindus. This
was because 'natives' functioned mostly under the influence of emotions unlike the Europeans.[61]

The overcrowded situation of the asylums often determined not only
the reasons for mental illness among men and women, but also the cause
of mortality amongst both sexes. For instance, according to Surgeon
R. Bird of the Dullunda Asylum, the percentage of deaths among men
at Dullunda Asylum in 1872 was 9, or a little more than double the
mortality among women.

Although men stayed in less crowded wards, mortality was higher
among them in comparison to women who usually had to put up with
more crowded surroundings in the asylums. Also, men were in a better
position than women, but even then mortality was higher amongst the
former. In 1872, 49 women were admitted as against 170 men. This

[60] Home Department, Medical B Proceedings, Number 80, July 1894,
'Report on Lunatic Asylums of Bengal for the Year 1893,' by H. Harvey,
Inspector General of Civil Hospitals, NAI.
[61] *Annual Report on the Insane Asylums of Bengal for the Year 1872*, by
J. Campbell Brown.

disproportion, it was believed, did not indicate that the male population was more liable to mental illness than the females, but only that
men afflicted with the disease were more readily brought to the asylum
than women. This owed partly to the custom of secluding women
which prevailed in India, and partly to women being more easily managed at home than the men.[62]

According to James Wise, Superintendent of Dacca Lunatic Asylum,
mental depression was very common among 'natives' and suicidal tendencies were often the consequence. Among those treated during the
past year (1872), one Muslim woman, three Hindu men, and one Hindu
woman had attempted to commit suicide before they were admitted.
Two Muslim and three Hindu men attempted to commit suicide since
they came to the asylum. The number of Muslims and Hindus who
committed suicide were almost equal. Over time, the number of patients
who committed suicide increased so much that between 1869 and 1872,
the bodies of twenty-seven Hindu and twenty-four Muslim men and
forty-nine Hindu and forty-five Muslim women, who committed suicide by hanging while temporarily insane, were sent to the police for
examination.[63]

According to James Wise, grief over the loss of children or parents
and anxiety were the most frequent moral causes of mental illness among
'natives'. Sixteen women out of a total of forty-six women admitted
at the Dacca Asylum during the year were reported as 'mad' due to
the loss of family members. Only 33 out of 214 males were affected
in a similar manner. Debauchery was understood as a moral cause of
insanity. James Wise in 1872 stated that intoxication alone was not the
cause of mental illness; rather, insanity was the result of a combination
of causes.

> The wild, reckless, and irregular life, and the feeling of self degradation, was
> probably more to do with the production of insanity than the sensuality and
> depravity of their lives.[64]

[62] *Annual Report on the Insane Asylums of Bengal for the Year 1872*, by
J. Campbell Brown.
[63] *Annual Report on the Insane Asylums of Bengal for the Year 1872*, by
J. Campbell Brown.
[64] James Wise, 'Report on Dacca Lunatic Asylum for 1872,' *Annual Report
on the Insane Asylums of Bengal for the Year 1872*.

In 1872, in the European Lunatic Asylum, the moral causes of insanity included pecuniary difficulties and domestic troubles. Of the four patients admitted in the asylum during the year, three men and one woman suffered from such moral causes. Five women died during childbirth. Amongst the rest of the women admitted during the year, there were instances of puerperal mania and imbecility. The uncertainty over the understanding of insanity was thus stated by the Superintendent:

> It was not to be understood that all cases could be so strictly classified with accuracy; for it was difficult in many cases to decide what name the disease should bear, and this for the reason, that the manifestations of the disease in many persons are characteristic of more than one variety. For instance, it was not easy to say in many cases whether the disease was chronic mania, or acute mania, for the time comparatively quiescent; chronic mania or dementia; chronic mania, with fixed delusion or melancholia, liable to lapse into mania. The nomenclature, in most instances, was only approximately correct.[65]

In 1884, one woman died of acute mania at the European Lunatic Asylum.[66] In 1890, the proportion of recoveries among the patients there was very low. This, according to the superintendent, was due to the admission of a greater number of women during the year. He further stated that women were found to suffer more frequently than men from the 'chronic' and 'incurable' forms of insanity.[67] The views of the medical practitioners in England about insane women were reflected while treating women at the European Lunatic Asylum. The medical officers considered the mental illness of European women as 'incurable', and probably held the same view for women in the 'native' asylums.

Most of the women in the 'native' lunatic asylums during 1862 suffered from mania and acute mania, with one or two cases of dementia or

[65] R. Bird, 'Report on the Bhawanipore Lunatic Asylum,' *Annual Report on the Insane Asylums of Bengal for the Year 1872*.

[66] Home Department, Medical Board Proceedings, Number 100, September 1885, 'Report on the Lunatic Asylums of Bengal for 1884,' by J. W. Edgar, Officiating Secretary to the Government of Bengal, NAI.

[67] Home Department, Medical Board Proceedings, Number 133, July 1890, 'Report on the Lunatic Asylums of Bengal for the Year 1889,' by C. Stevens, Officiating Chief Secretary to the Government of Bengal, NAI.

monomania and melancholia (see Tables 3.4 and 3.5).[68] Mania or monomania was not restricted to women, many male patients also suffered from it. In fact, the report of the Patna Lunatic Asylum showed that there were more cases of mania among men than among female lunatics (see Table 3.6). A. Fleming stated that the cause of insanity for most of the patients at the Mooshedabad Asylum was dysentery and consumption of ganja and liquor. The reason why many of the patients were admitted in a weak and debilitated condition to the asylum was because they belonged to the poorest section of society. He further stated that none of the 'better' classes were willing to send the patient for treatment at the asylum; instead, they preferred to treat them in their own ways at home.[69] Therefore, both men and women suffered from the similar causes of insanity. However, some of the medical officers tried to make a distinction in understanding the insanity of women as separate from that of men.

According to J. Fullarton, of the moral causes, grief, particularly amongst women, was the principal cause of mental illness in the asylums of Bengal in 1876. Next in 'order' were anger, religion, poverty, and love, which were also considered important reasons for insanity among women. Of the total number of women treated in the asylums of Bengal, 45.73 per cent suffered from mental illnesses due to physical causes, 7.93 per cent from moral causes, and 46.33 per cent from unknown causes.[70] According to Superintendent Payne of the Dullunda Asylum, dysentery, fever, diseases of the nervous system, and phthisis, covered 60 per cent of the total admissions among the male patients, while among the women, diseases of the nervous system, dysentery, cholera, and fevers contributed more than half of the admissions.[71] He further stated that another very troublesome affliction among women, whose cause and prevention was a problem to be solved, was the presence of a large

[68] A. Simpson, 'Report on the Dacca Lunatic Asylum for the Year 1862,' *Annual Reports and Returns of the Insane Asylums in Bengal for the year 1862*, compiled by J. McClelland, Officiating Principal Inspector General, Medical Department (Calcutta: Military Orphan Press, 1863), NAI.

[69] A. Fleming, 'Report on the Moorshedabad Lunatic Asylum for the Year 1862'.

[70] *Annual Report on the Insane Asylums of Bengal for the Year 1876*, by J. Fullarton Beatson.

[71] *Annual Report on the Insane Asylums of Bengal for the Year 1876*, by J. Fullarton Beatson.

Table 3.4 Cases of Monomania, Imbecility, Dementia, and Melancholia among Female Inmates at Dullunda Asylum during the Year 1862

Name	Age	Occupation	Caste	Birth place	Diseases	Cause	Cause of death
Omourto	63	Unknown	H	Bengal	Mania Chronic	Unknown	
Belatone	42	,,	M	,,	,,	,,	Asthenia
Murtoo	33	,,	H	,,	,,	,,	
Jeerah	42	,,	M	,,	Monomania	,,	
Sallee	40	,,	CH	,,	Mania Acute	,,	
Manee	50	,,	,,	,,	Dementia	,,	
Dooknee or Peerun	32	,,	M	,,	Mania Chronic	,,	
Petteme, prisoner	43	,,	H	,,	,,	,,	Dysentery
Unknown, Boba	32	,,	,,	,,	,,	,,	
Kameenee or Rajee	26	,,	,,	,,	,,	,,	
Purressmonee	38	,,	,,	,,	,,	,,	Asthenia
Taree Kouranee	26	,,	,,	,,	,,	,,	
Jeebnee or Jhannobee	35	,,	,,	,,	,,	,,	
Sonah	50	,,	M	,,	,,	,,	Asthenia
Cowsullah	27	,,	H	,,	,,	,,	
Armon	43	,,	M	,,	,,	,,	Dysentery
Pecohree	50	,,	H	,,	,,	,,	
Dookee	25	,,	,,	,,	,,	,,	
Deenoe or Joymonee	40	,,	,,	,,	,,	,,	

(*Cont'd*)

Table 3.4 (*Cont'd*)

Name	Age	Occupation	Caste	Birth place	Diseases	Cause	Cause of death
Topsee	15	,,	CH	,,	,,	,,	
Doorgee	23	,,	H	,,	,,	,,	
Unknown, Surfee	33	,,	,,	,,	,,	,,	
Monglah, prisoner	25	,,	,,	,,	,,	,,	
Rushnee	27	,,	M	,,	Mania Acute	,,	
Talleeoh	30	,,	H	,,	Mania Chronic	,,	
Rossmonee	25	,,	M	,,	Mania Acute	,,	
Mulleeka	50	,,	H	,,	Mania Chronic	,,	
Hosainee	30	,,	M	,,	Mania Acute	,,	
Norkish	22	,,	CH	,,	Imbecility	,,	
Neemee	35	Juggee	H	,,	Dementia	,,	
Unknown, Number 39	35	Unknown	,,	,,	Melancholia	,,	Dysentery
Ahnah	30	,,	M	,,,,	Mania Acute	,,	Dysentery
Sumputee	60	,,	,,	,,	Melancholia	,,	Asthenia
Unknown, Number 44	40	,,	,,	,,	Dementia	,,	
Ullungo	28	,,	H	,,	Mania Acute	,,	Asthenia
Rammonee	35	,,	,,	,,	,,	,,	Dysentery
Surjee	30	,,	,,	,,	Imbecility	,,	
Beemolah or Beemoh	18	,,	M	,,	Mania Acute	,,	
Beendoo	40	,,	H	,,	,,	,,	

Name	Age			Diagnosis	Cause	Outcome
Asseemum	35	"	M	Mania Chronic	"	"
Gholabee	18	"	H	Mania Acute	"	Diarrhoea
Unknown, Soorjee, Number 47	28	"	"	Melancholia	"	"
Luchmonee	34	"	M	Mania Acute	"	Diarrhoea
Mohorum	30	"	"	Mania Chronic	Ganja Smg.	"
Tarramonee	30	"	H	Mania Acute	Unknown	Asthenia
Showba	30	"	"	"	"	"
Buckee	35	"	"	Mania Chronic	"	"
Bissasee	10	"	CH	Amentia	"	"
Obhoyoh	40	"	M	Mania Acute	Congenital	"
Kissorree	30	"	H	"	Unknown	"
Settah Raur	30	"	"	"	Ganja Smg.	"
Assoorun	50	"	M	"	"	Dysentery
Parbutty	35	"	H	"	"	"
Alladee	25	"	"	"	Unknown	"
Mungaun	50	"	M	"	"	Asthenia
Rannee	38	"	H	Mania Chronic	Ganja Smg.	"
Saddee	30	"	"	Mania Acute	Unknown	"
Rannee	38	"	"	Mania Chronic	Ganja Smg.	Dysentery
Rushnee, alias Sugnee	30	"	"	Mania Acute	Unknown	"

Source: 'Annual Returns of 'Native' Female Insane Patients Treated in the Asylum at Dullunda during the Year 1862' in *Annual Reports and Returns of the Insane Asylums in Bengal*, compiled by J. McClelland (Calcutta: Military Orphan Press, 1863), NAI.

Table 3.5 Cases of Mania among Female Inmates at the Moorshedabad Asylum during the Year 1862

Name (Females)	Age	Religion or Caste	Birthplace, Village, Purgunnah or Zilla	Diseases	Cause
Shooroo Dunnee	37	H	Rajshaye	Dementia	Unknown
Doyamoye Kashobe	30	M	Rungpore	Mania	Unknown
Ameer Buksheee	30	M	Bhaugulpore	Mania	Unknown
Name Unknown	55	H	Burdwan	Mania	Unknown
Pualee	32	M	Rungpore	Mania	Unknown
Ameerun Beva	55	M	Moorshedabad	Mania	Unknown
Dasi	30	M	Moorshedabad	Mania	Unknown
Name Unknown	30	M	Burdwan	Mania	Unknown
Alladee P.	38	M	Bheerbhoom	Dementia	Unknown

Source: A. Fleming, 'Report on the Moorshedabad Lunatic Asylum for the Year 1862,' *Annual Report and Returns of Insane Asylums in Bengal for the year 1863* (Calcutta: Military Orphan Press, 1863), NAI.

Table 3.6 Different Types of Insanity among Men and Women, Patna Lunatic Asylum, 1862

	Male	Female	Total
Mania	24	6	30
Dementia	8	1	9
Amentia	1	0	1
Moral Insanity	0	0	0
Monomania	0	0	0
Total	33	7	40

Source: *Annual Reports and Returns of the Insane Asylums in Bengal for the year 1862*, compiled by J. McClelland, Officiating Principal Inspector General, Medical Department (Calcutta: Military Orphan Press, 1863), NAI.

quantity of intestinal roundworms. This sometimes caused fatal injury, and at times it became a source of perplexity.[72]

[72] *Annual Report on the Insane Asylums of Bengal for the Year 1876*, by J. Fullarton Beatson.

John Haslam, who was in charge of several madhouses in England, stated that insanity was more frequent among men than women. Women, according to him, were more prone to mental illness because of certain natural processes that they undergo, such as menstruation, parturition, and preparing nutriment for the infant, along with certain diseases which they suffered from during those times.[73] His view was refuted by J. Swiney of the Medical Board in India. According to him, Haslam's views were applicable for understanding female insanity in England, but it was difficult to assume the same in case of 'native' women in India. He further stated that

> our want of more general seclusion of females adopted in this country precludes our getting correct information or making an accurate comparison upon this point but the females who are admitted into our presidency insane hospital are few in number as compared with the males.[74]

Following Swiney's comment it could be concluded that in England, not only were case histories of patients regularly maintained after admission, but most patients were also admitted along with a prior case history. But in India this was not possible. Most of the patients admitted in the 'native' asylums in Bengal mainly belonged to the poorer sections of society. They were not always admitted by their friends, family, or relatives. In many cases, they were also picked up from the street by *chowkidar*s or policemen. Therefore, it was difficult to state whether insanity was more frequent among men than among women in India. Swiney did not look at mental illness as a consequence of pain or mere suffering, but as the 'independent and associated effects of the general diseases'. Although he yielded that it was difficult to conclude anything 'in our present state of contracted knowledge' about insanity, he could not ignore that 'mental functions may possibly be disturbed by similar causes to those which disturb the bodily functions'.[75]

[73] Medical Board Proceedings, Number 8, Enclosure to Letter from Mr Swiney to James Hutchinson, 24 March 1835.

[74] Medical Board Proceedings, Number 8, Enclosure to Letter from Mr Swiney to James Hutchinson, 24 March 1835.

[75] Medical Board Proceedings, Number 8, Enclosure to Letter from Mr Swiney to James Hutchinson, 24 March 1835.

To further understand the causes of mental illness among women, it is important to take into consideration some of the case studies from the period. Based on the condition of women admitted to the asylums and their case histories, this study is divided into two categories: first, insanity amongst women in the European Lunatic Asylum, and second, the condition of women admitted in the 'native' asylums of Bengal.

WOMEN IN THE EUROPEAN LUNATIC ASYLUM

Delirium, one of the causes of mental illness, was dealt by practitioners at the asylum, but complete recovery from it was usually not reported. While the doctors could diagnose its symptoms, they did not have the expertise during the early nineteenth century to treat the problem. Such was the case of an orphaned child named Eliza Wallace. She was the daughter of a Sergeant in His Majesty's 22nd Regiment and was admitted to the Insane Hospital in Calcutta on 29 March 1810.[76] At the age of five she was sent to the Hospital from Berhampore Cantonment. Eliza, according to medical officers, suffered from delirium since her childhood. Her father's death affected her very badly and worsened her situation. Members of the regiment could not take care of her any more, as delirium needed special attention.[77] The Lieutenant Colonel, under whose supervision Eliza's father had served, took an initiative to pay for her well-being and maintenance from the allowance granted by the East India Company.[78] But, gradually as her situation worsened, she was sent to the Insane Hospital in Calcutta for further treatment, under the expenses of the Company.

[76] Medical Board Proceedings, March 1810, Letter sent to Dr Fleming, First Member of the Medical Board from Alexander Russell, Surgeon to the Hospital for Insane, dated 29 March 1810, NAI.

[77] Medical Board Proceedings, February 1810, Letter sent to Commanding Officer, His Majesty's 22 Foot, Colonel Dalrymple from Major E. Lindsay, dated 21 February 1810.

[78] Medical Board Proceedings, February 1810, Letter sent to Lieutenant Colonel W. G. Heir to Commanding Officer, His Majesty's 22 Foot, Colonel Dalrymple, dated 27 January 1810, NAI.

A person with a 'deranged mind' was also considered insane. However, such a state of mind was never very clearly outlined by the doctors. Usually, patients with such diagnoses were held at the asylum for a short period, but not all of them were released early. The medical officers were hopeful with such patients as they thought that a 'deranged mind' could be 'cured and discharged if treated on time'. For instance, Mrs Adam, wife of Sergeant Adam of His Majesty's 14th Foot Regiment, was admitted to the Hospital on 7 October 1810. When admitted she was diagnosed with a 'deranged mind'. But, within three weeks she was diagnosed as completely cured and was ordered to be discharged from the Hospital by the medical examiners.[79]

In another instance, Mrs Gopert was admitted in a state of derangement to the Insane Hospital in Calcutta on 13 April 1813 by her husband Captain Gopert of the country service.[80] For a period of one year, her husband paid for her expenses until he went on an assignment in command of a ship and thenceforth the asylum did not receive any news from him. In his absence she was taken care of by the Surgeon of the Hospital, who paid for her treatment from his own expenses. In 1816, the Surgeon appealed to the Medical Board to relieve him from the charges. He expressed his concern for her 'unhappy' state. As she had no relatives or friends to take care of her, the Surgeon requested the Board to take the help of the government for her maintenance at the asylum. Mrs Gopert's 'derangement' was described by the Surgeon as violent and unmanageable. He further stated that Mrs Gopert was a 'Gentlewoman', which he concluded from her 'habits' and 'education'. Therefore, according to him, it would neither be 'proper nor humane to place her on the footing of the lower class of patients'.[81] The Medical Board, in a letter to the Chief Secretary to Government,

[79] Medical Board Proceedings, December 1810, Letter sent to Surgeon Russell at the Hospital for Insane from I. Fleming, First Member of the Medical Board, NAI.

[80] Medical Board Proceedings, February 1813, Letter sent to Dr Monro, First Member Medical Board from Robert Leny, Surgeon Insane Hospital, Calcutta, dated 14 April 1813, NAI.

[81] Medical Board Proceedings, August 1816, Letter sent to Peter Cochrane, First Member Medical Board from Robert Leny, Surgeon, Insane Hospital Calcutta, dated 6 August 1816, NAI.

requested Mrs Gopert to be maintained as an upper-class patient.[82] She was described as 'violent and unmanageable'. In this instance, as in the previous one, the question of her expenses was well taken care of.

Another cause of insanity was melancholia. Major Greene, the Commanding Artillery of Chunar Garrison died leaving behind Mrs Greene in a state of 'distrust and melancholy' from which she had been suffering for a long time. The suregeon of the garrison, in a letter to the Board, requested them to admit her into the asylum at Calcutta. The Surgeon, who was also in charge of Major Greene's last will, stated that the whole of his property was bequeathed to his wife after the payment of his debts. But the Surgeon was anxious that not much would be left after paying off the debts and there was little probability of anything being saved. However, it was settled that regular accounts of the property would be paid and whatever remained would also be paid to the Board if they were willing to admit her to the asylum at Calcutta.[83] The Medical Board was of the opinion that upon her arrival in Calcutta, she should not be admitted to the Insane Hospital of Calcutta by her friends under any circumstances. Instead, she should be admitted to the House of Reception, privately owned by Mr Bearsdmore. Although Europeans were temporarily admitted to the Insane Hospital of Calcutta before they were shifted to either the House of Reception or sent back to England, it was not considered by the Medical Board to be a proper place of admission 'for females of respectable condition in life, and of delineate habits'.[84] The Medical Board took the initiative to establish the Insane Hospital of Calcutta, and they were responsible for the 'natives' admitted there. However, when it came to admitting Europeans, they considered the asylum completely unsuitable, more so if the patient belonged to the upper class of society. Both the economic factor, which included due

[82] Medical Board Proceedings, August 1816, Letter sent to C. M. Ricketts, Chief Secretary to Government from Peter Cochrane, First Member Medical Board, dated 8 August 1816, NAI.

[83] Medical Board Proceedings, Number 53, 28 September 1820, Letter sent to James Jameson, Secretary Medical Board from G. Playfair, Garrison Surgeon, Chunar, dated 6 September 1820, NAI.

[84] Medical Board Proceedings, Number 54, 28 September 1820, Letter sent to G. Playfair, Garrison Surgeon, Chunar from J. Jameson, Secretary Medical Board, Medical Board Office, dated 15 September 1820, NAI.

payment of patients, and racial prejudices were important for a European patient's admission into an asylum. The government benefitted from the paying-in patients who primarily belonged to the upper classes, as those payments helped the government to maintain the establishment, thereby reducing its financial pressure. Therefore, the Board requested the Garrison Surgeon of Chunar to send an account of Mrs Green's economic condition, which included any sort of property or income, so that it might be used for her maintenance at the House of Reception. The Board also asked for a 'certificate of insanity' signed by two medical officers to be submitted to the Surgeon of the asylum at the time of her admission.

The case studies of three women—Mrs Margaret Northon, Ketty Barlow, and Fatima—at Beardsmore's House of Reception in 1821 and the issues related to their discharge after cure are discussed in the following section. Mrs Margaret Northon was a half-caste woman. She was the widow of a quartermaster sergeant in the Bengal army who had died about eighteen years earlier. She did not have friends. The problem with her case was that she appeared to be perfectly sane during winter, but the malady aggravated during the summer when she was diagnosed 'silly' and 'helpless'. According to Margaret, she was admitted into the Insane Hospital by a conductor named Hunter. In another instance, the case of Ketty Barlow, a Portuguese woman, widow of a person who was formerly in the service of a Colonel Smith, was different. She was admitted because she had 'frequent attacks', although she was never violent. The reason for Barlow's 'frequent attacks' could be epileptic seizures, although no such entry was made in the report. At the time of her admission, she was known to have a son, who was an assistant to an indigo planter in the Burdwan district of Bengal. But over time, her son had abandoned her and the asylum officers did not receive any further information about his whereabouts. Therefore, her maintenance at the asylum became a serious cause of concern for the administrators. The third patient was Fatima, a Malay girl who was sent to the asylum from Mrs Marshmans' School in Serampore. She was diagnosed as an 'idiot', but not mischievous.[85] After the abolition of the Insane Hospital at

[85] Medical Board Proceedings, Number 15, 13 January 1821, Letter sent to C. Lushington, Secretary to Government in General Department from James Jameson, Secretary Medical Board, dated Medical Board Office, 12 January 1821, NAI.

Calcutta, these three women were transferred to Mr Beardsmore's House for temporary reception, and, in the event of their not recovering in time, ultimately destined for Europe. The problem faced under such circumstances was that it was not possible to maintain them in the private asylum. On the Board's order to remove them to the European Asylum or to the Insane Hospital maintained by the government, Mrs Northon refused to go and it was mutually decided between her and Mr Beardsmore, the proprietor of the House of Reception, that she would stay back in the asylum and take the position of one of the keepers of the asylum. The Board proposed the removal of two other female patients to the Insane Hospital at Russapaglah.[86] Under the rules of the European Insane Hospital, patients who were finally sent back to England were admitted there. But Fatima and Ketty Barlow did not have European connections, and, hence, they had no place for admission in the European Lunatic Asylum. Consequently, in a letter to Mr Beardsmore, the Board confirmed Mrs Northon's stay at the House of Reception and ordered for the immediate removal of two patients to Russapaglah,[87] who were then maintained by the government. The case of Margaret Northon was a classic case of illness determined by the tropical weather condition. The climatic condition of India was often conveniently interpreted by European physicians as a reason for mental illness in the country. For instance, this argument was substantiated by W. A. Green of Dacca, when in 1857, he stated:

> Insanity among natives of India and the East is probably as frequent if not more so, than in the temperate and colder climates of other parts of the world.[88]

The case of Ketty Barlow was an intriguing one as symptoms of her illness were approved by the medical officers on the basis of a narration

[86] Medical Board Proceedings, Number 15, Letter from James Jameson to C. Lushington, 12 January 1821.

[87] Medical Board Proceedings, Number 8, 19 February 1821, Letter sent to Mr Beardsmore, Proprietor, Lunatic Asylum from J. Jameson, Secretary Medical Board, Medical Board Office, dated 14 February 1821, NAI.

[88] W A Greene, 'Contributions towards the Pathology of Insanity in India,' The Annals of Medical Science, 4 (1857): 375, WL.

made by a non-medical person. Therefore, it is important here to note how a non-professional person understood symptoms of mental illness, and also how a medically certified insane person perceived it. In a letter sent to the Secretary of Medical Board, W. Senior, an army man, expressed his concern about Katherine Barlow (Ketty). Katherine, or Ketty Barlow as he addressed her, was the childhood friend of his wife. This army man's wife even nursed her when she was unwell. Based on his observations, he emphasized that she was not only in full possession of her reason but was also harmless. Her aberration originated from a thought within her mind that 'her property was stolen'. She also narrated 'absurd tales' of which she was the heroine. He further stated that she had lived a better life while she was employed as a French teacher in a school in England.[89] The telling of absurd tales was not necessarily seen by her friends as a cause of her insanity. While he narrated her life to state that she was not 'mad' but somebody who needed little care and attention to get back to the normal course of life, the same narration became a significant cause of concern for the medical practitioners who considered those reasons enough for her to be defined as an insane person who needed treatment. W. Senior further stated that the 'poor woman's' well-being was more likely to be ensured when she was placed in the institution, than when entrusted to the care of an individual. He was anxious that at the asylum she would not have a companion to dance or sing with or narrate her 'little tales' of life to and would die of a broken heart. Hence, he requested the Board to look into her case with care and concern during her stay at the asylum.[90]

Europeans were sent back to England after a short stay at the asylum. It was considered by the medical practitioners that further improvement was not possible in India because of the climatic conditions. Similarly, the Medical Board decided to send Mrs Ann Hartley back home after her stay at the European Insane Hospital for a period of approximately three months from November 1820. She was not

[89] Medical Board Proceedings, Number 15, 19 February 1821, Letter sent to James Jameson, Secretary Medical Board from W. Senior, Lieutenant First Battalion Tenth Regiment Native Infantry, dated 16 February 1821, NAI.

[90] Medical Board Proceedings, Number 15, Letter from W. Senior to James Jameson, 16 February 1821.

cured and was sent out with many other 'lunatic' men on the ship *Mary*.[91] She was accommodated on the ship in a separate cabin because of her violent and refractory nature, along with a female keeper. Mrs Hartley was the widow of a soldier. Nothing was known of her birth or parentage. She was violent and had a tendency to hurt herself.[92] She had two children. One child was with her in the asylum and the other was admitted to the Orphan School. Once her journey back home was finalized, the Board decided to separate the second child from her as well and admit her at the Orphan School in Calcutta, as she was entitled to get the benefits which the orphan of a soldier in the Company's army was fully entitled to.[93]

In another similar instance of the patient being sent back to England, the Medical Board stated that Mrs Pollard was ready to board the ship to return to England for further treatment in January 1829.[94] The case history prepared during her stay in the asylum was also sent to England. It stated Mrs Pollard was a person of choleric temperament. She was of middle stature and was very stout. Her exact age was not known and it was assumed that she was between 30 to 40 years of age. She had been addicted to spirituous liquors since the death of her husband. This 'propensity becoming a confirmed habit she exhibited symptoms of madness'. She was sent to the asylum from the Upper Provinces of India. During her admission in February 1828, she exhibited an appearance of complete 'idiocy', laughing and crying alternately and talking in a most silly and incoherent manner. Mrs Pollard's propensity for drinking was on her mind, but she did

[91] Medical Board Proceedings, Number 14, 12 February 1821, Letter sent to C. Lushington, Secretary to Government in General Department from James Jameson, Secretary Medical Board, NAI.

[92] Medical Board Proceedings, Number 14, Enclosure attached to Letter from James Jameson to C. Lushington.

[93] Medical Board Proceedings, Number 39, 14 February 1821, Letter sent to Mr J. Sawers, Surgeon, Insane Hospital from James Jameson, Secretary Medical Board, NAI.

[94] Medical Board Proceedings, Number 9, 2 February 1829, Letter sent to T. Princep, Secretary to Government in General Department from J. Adam, Secretary Medical Board, Medical Board Office, dated 24 January 1829, NAI.

not dwell long on the thought as she could not obtain it. Her physical health improved as the condition of her mind improved, but she continued to remain 'silly and imbecile'. She occasionally complained of a headache and was administered with the required dosage of purgatives for constipation. Almost a year later, by January 1829, she was diagnosed as perfectly tranquil.[95] She was married to one Mr Pollard in India regarding whom the Board had no information either. She had seven sisters, all of whom were settled in England, but did not have any relatives or friends in India. But her sisters, relatives, and friends never tried to contact her.[96]

Mary Mac Donald, wife of John Mac Donald of the Corps in Dinapore Division, was sent to the European Asylum from Dinapore with an escort of a sepoy and two female European attendants. Her medical case history was prepared by Surgeon J. Mouat. This was sent to the officers of the Medical Board.[97] Mary Mac Donald was twenty-eight years old. She had lived in India for only a year before her admission. She was of a melancholic temperament and had a 'wild and peculiar look' on her face. She was found in a state of 'mental derangement' since she had disembarked from the ship in 1827. Following that time she was often 'violent and outrageous'. Hence, she was frequently taken to the General Hospital for medical treatment by her family members. Finally, on 10 February 1829, when she was admitted into the hospital at Dinapore, she had a 'wild staring look', and great loquacity, but all expressed with an incoherency of speech. According to her husband, she was frequently 'deranged' and violent at home. On admission her pulse beat was counted to be 130, her face was often flushed, and her 'wild look' got worse due to the effect of vine sections, purgatives, and calomel. She got better and was discharged on 3 March 1829, but again readmitted

[95] Medical Board Proceedings, Number 9, Letter from J. Adam to T. Princep, 24 January 1829.

[96] Medical Board Proceedings, Number 7, 16 March 1829, Letter sent to C. B. Greenlaw, Secretary Marine Board from John Adam, Secretary Medical Board, Medical Board Office, dated 12 March 1829, NAI.

[97] Medical Board Proceedings, 8 June 1829, Letter sent to J. Adam, Secretary Medical Board from A. Cameron, Lieutenant Colonel Commanding Buffs, dated 1 June 1829, NAI.

on 7 March in a most violent and delirious state. Since then she was either in a sullen mood, occasionally answering questions asked by the doctors, or expressing absolute rationality of thought, although her countenance did not lose its wild and peculiar look. She was made to bleed with leeches placed on her head; cold effusions were applied, blisters were made on the head and neck as it made the patients less irritable, and powerful purgatives like calomel were applied to affect the mouth. A straitjacket was used to restrain her. All this gave her 'temporary relief', and after being quiet and rational for five or six days she became loquacious and violent again. During that phase, she destroyed her clothes, disturbed other patients, and endeavoured to set fire to the hospital. From the repeated relapses and the peculiar wild look, Surgeon J. Mouat, under whose treatment she was admitted in the hospital, considered her almost incurable. She was considered unfit to remain in Dinapore any longer. Moreover, according to the Surgeon, she could have been dangerous if left behind in the barracks.[98] Melancholia was perhaps considered one of the most common causes of mental illness. Given that its symptoms recurred in frequent intervals, a longer treatment under observation in a specialized and confined place was considered suitable by the medical practitioners of the time. Hence, they were sent to the asylums.

Mrs M. Gammon was admitted as a public patient at Mr Beardsmore's private asylum in 1835 on the recommendation of Dr Hutchinson, Secretary to the Medical Board. She was of European origin and was sent from the 28th Regiment. Nothing was known of her husband but it could be assumed that he worked as an officer at the Regiment. At the time of her admission, she was diagnosed with amnesia. Gradually, Gammon's mental condition improved; she appeared cheerful, happy, and in good health.[99] On the evening of 1 April 1836, she delivered a male child. She regained her usual health and strength and occasionally nursed her child. But at certain moments of irrational lapses she threw the child out of her arms. Under such circumstances the asylum staff

[98] Medical Board Proceeding, 8 June 1829, Letter sent to A. Cameron, Lieutenant Colonel Commanding Buffs, from J. Mouat, Surgeon of His Majesty's Buffs, Bhagulpore, dated 24 May 1829, NAI.

[99] General Proceedings, General Department, Number 35, October 1835, Monthly Return of Public Patients at Beardsmore's Asylum, WBSA.

intervened. Her baby was put in the care of a nurse. The superintendent of the asylum reported that her mental health did not improve 'because she gave birth'.[100] The child was finally separated from her and was admitted at the Lower Orphan School of Calcutta.[101]

As payment was mandatory for patients at the European Lunatic Asylum, failure to do so affected the fate of lunatics. In the case of women like Miss Eliza Ross, even though she was initially admitted as a first-class patient at the European Lunatic Asylum, she was later shifted to the category of 'public patient' because, after the death of her partner, Captain Ross, she did not have anyone to pay for her maintenance. Along with ill-health, this transfer in the category of patients caused further difficulties as the arrangements for a first-class patient in an asylum were very different from that of public patients. The report of 1850 stated that she had been at the asylum for a long time. According to the Board, the relationship between Eliza and Captain Ross gave her no claim to support from him. Captain Ross, a marine store keeper at Khiderpore, in Calcutta, had a family to look after. Because of his sudden death, no provision was arranged either for his family or for Miss Eliza Ross. Hence, under such circumstances the Board decided to transfer her to the category of public patients.[102]

There were also instances when relatives wanted to take patients back home for further treatment and care. In 1850, this happened in the case of Mrs Pearson, a patient at the Bhawanipore Lunatic Asylum. Her sister, Mrs Taylor, was able to convince the Board that they were in a position to ensure to her suitable professional treatment at home and all the humane care that the she required.[103]

---

[100] General Proceedings, General Department, Number 29, 13 April 1836, Report on the Public Patients Admitted at Beardsmore's Asylum by the Superintendent Mr Beardsmore, WBSA.

[101] General Proceedings, General Department, Number 17, 20 April 1836, Report on the Public Patients admitted at Beardsmore's Asylum by the Superintendent Mr Beardsmore, WBSA.

[102] Medical Board Proceedings, Number 15, 2 May 1850, Letter sent to the Governor of Bengal from the Medical Board Office, dated 29 April 1850, NAI.

[103] Medical Board Proceedings, Number 9, 26 December 1850, Letter sent to Mrs Sims, Proprietor of Bhawanipore Lunatic Asylum from Dr Forsyth, Secretary Medical Board, dated 23 December 1850, NAI.

CASE STUDIES OF SOME OF THE 'NATIVE' WOMEN

This section contains certain case histories of patients admitted at Dacca Asylum during 1842. The situation at the 'native' asylum was very different from that of the European Asylum. A couple of case histories discussed here show how insanity of women was understood by the medical officers and what kind of treatment was provided to cure them.

Mussumat Ropee, was admitted on 2 January at the age of fifty-six. She was of the *chandal* caste, and a beggar. Her history, prior to her admission at the hospital, was unknown. At the asylum, she usually sat in a corner of her apartment and avoided interaction with other patients. She spoke wildly and incoherently, and frequently addressed 'imaginary persons' in the room. She was monitored with regular dosages of aperients and tonics.

Mussumat Omrah was admitted at the age of thirty on 22 January. She used to sit idly in her house and refused to eat. She was apparently in a state of deep melancholy prior to her admission to the hospital. She attempted to set fire to a house after which she was sent to the thana and then to the asylum. She was epileptic and had four attacks in a day since her admission to the hospital. She also had recurrent fever and bilious diarrhoea. Her catamenia was regular. She gradually became weak and emaciated. Tonics including nitrates of silver were administered. Following a series of epileptic seizures, she went into a coma and died on 15 December. While going through similar cases, at a much later period in 1872, the superintendent of the Moydapore Asylum also administered dosage of nitrate of silver in one to three grains daily with asafoetida for the treatment of epilepsy. It was expected that such doses would effectually control the attacks and cure the case.[104] Therefore, while epilepsy was treated, her melancholia, fever, and diarrhoea were not taken into consideration.

Catamenia, or the regular flow of menstrual cycle, often determined the understanding of a woman's insanity. According to the physicians, as long as a woman's menstrual cycle was regular, they expected her recovery. This understanding of women's insanity was also seen in other case studies. Elaine Showalter had pointed out that 'doctors argued that

---

[104] J. M. Coates, 'Report on the Moydapore Lunatic Asylum for the Year 1872,' *Annual Report on the Insane Asylums of Bengal for the Year 1872.*

the menstrual discharge in itself predisposed women to insanity. Either an abnormal quantity or quality of the blood, according to this theory, could affect the brain. Therefore, physicians attempted to control the blood by diet and venesection.'[105]

It was often considered by the medical practitioners that anxiety might lead to insanity. For instance, Mussumat Maunne, a twine maker who was admitted on 3 February at the age of forty, was diagnosed with anxiety on admission. The cause of her anxiety was her son-in-law who was wounded and whom a 'native' physician had failed to cure. On her admission to the hospital, she spoke incoherently and was inclined to be violent. She was filthy in her habits. She wandered in the garden and talked to herself. Her catamenia was regular. A tartar emetic solution was administered to her, but she showed little signs of improvement. She was administered with regular dosages of purgatives and camphor mixture. Unlike the case studies of European 'lunatic' women during 1810 to early 1830s, by 1840s there were instances of medical interference, where constant experiments were made with pills and their dosage.

Mussumat Alta was admitted on 5 February, at the age of forty. She was the wife of a cultivator. She was very violent at the time of her admission. She tore her clothes and blankets into shreds. Her tongue was foul, which indicated a diseased secretion. Tartar emetic solutions and purgatives were prescribed. Her catamenia was irregular. She was given dosages of aloetic and myrrh pills. Aloetic pills were made of aloe, a plant, mainly used as purgatives, and myrrh helped in healing wounds and ulcers. Her catamenia became regular by 16 July. From the moment her menstrual cycle became regular, the physicians concluded that she had begun to improve. She was noticed to be quiet, often amusing herself by picking up straw and pieces of bricks. She was subsequently employed in asylum labour: arranging the bedding of the patients, carrying their dinner from the cook room, and cleaning dishes. She was discharged as cured on 17 December.

A nineteen-year-old prostitute, Mussumat Anundo, was admitted on 5 March. Anundo was sent from Mymensingh. She was admitted at the asylum as she showed 'symptoms of insanity' like abusing people at her locality. She was found wandering around the countryside when

[105] Showalter, *The Female Malady*, 56.

she was picked up by the police. On her admission, she indulged in immoderate fits of singing, crying, and dancing. She tore her clothes into pieces. Her catamenia was suppressed. Aloetic and myrrh pills were prescribed to her. Her menstruation recommenced on 22 May and she began to improve. During her convalescence she spun thread, cleaned cotton, and occasionally amused herself. She was discharged as cured on 25 September.

Mrs Marion George Panioty was sixty years old. She was a Greek woman. She was removed to the asylum after a representation was made to the Magistrate about the miserable condition in which she was kept by her relatives in town. She was found in a low damp cellar or godown and from her emaciated appearance, she looked as as though she had been starving. In the asylum she was quiet and harmless, although dirty in her habits. She was emaciated and stooped from disability and age. On admission she suffered from diarrhoea, which continued for almost a month, for which astringents and tonics were prescribed. The treatment failed. She was removed from the hospital by her friends on 23 May and died the same evening.

Amonee, a Hindu, was admitted on 26 March at the age of twenty. She was sent from Assam. She was 'noisy' and made frequent attempts to escape from the hospital. She became violent, tore her clothes, and destroyed or injured whatever or whosoever was found near her. She was even inclined to strike female attendants. Her catamenia was regular. She talked a lot, but in a language that neither the doctors nor the asylum attendants could follow. She was occasionally employed in asylum labour; worked at the *dhenkee*,[106] swept the compound, and picked cotton. Amonee was administered with occasional dosages of purgatives, which showed gradual improvement in her health.

Fyzun, a Muslim, was admitted on 28 March at the age of thirty-five. She was from the *meerasen* caste. Fyzun was addicted to ganja. She molested and abused her neighbours and stole their property without attempting to conceal it. She was under the impression that it was her own. She rolled about on the ground when admitted into hospital, and tore off her clothes. She also threw fits of violent rage. Her catamenia was regular. Her general health was good. She became convalescent since the middle of August from the time she was employed to work at the

[106] A pounding instrument used in villages to produce huskless paddy.

dhenkee. She swept the compound and wards, and arranged the bedding and clothing of the female patients. She was discharged as cured on 24 October.

Mussumat Komalle was admitted to the hospital on 12 April. She was thirty-five years old and was from the chandal caste. Komalle was a prostitute. Before her admission at the asylum, she was under medical treatment at the Native Hospital for a bowel complaint where she was diagnosed with symptoms of 'mental derangement'. Those symptoms were singing, talking to herself, and annoying other patients by seizing their bedding and clothes. On admission she became dull and languid and was disinclined to move or speak. Her catamenia was irregular. Aloetic and myrrh pills were prescribed to her. Menstruation commenced on 1 June and since then a gradual improvement in her health was noticed. She was employed at dhenkee and finally discharged as cured on 17 May.

Mussumat Utter was admitted on 29 March. She was forty years old. She was the wife of a cultivator. Utter was found by the police wandering about abusing and ill-treating people. She was 'exceedingly noisy and turbulent' on her admission. Utter tore off her clothes and attempted to strike any person who approached her. She had the habit of besmearing her body with mud. She broke out at times into fits of great excitement. Her catamenia was regular. She had fallen and broken her arms about six months earlier, but gradually recovered from it. There was little or no permanent improvement in her case. She showed some symptoms of improvement since the beginning of September but had since then relapsed into her former condition. An emetic was administered on her admission. Purgatives were given to her at intervals.

Mussumat Ioynaul, a Muslim, was admitted on 18 May. She was thirty-five years old. The first indication of her insanity was her wandering about the town and abusing her neighbours. At times she would be excited and violent. Her catamenia was regular. She had been improving since the month of June. Ioynaul was rational in her conversation. She worked at the dhenkee. She was visited by her mother, and discharged after some time.

Mussumat Autter, a Muslim, was admitted on 9 June. She was the wife of Dengoo, a cultivator. She first showed symptoms of insanity when she began abusing her neighbours without any provocation, and at other times by observing obstinate silence and refusing to speak. On her admission into the asylum, she indulged in immoderate fits of laughter, made wry faces at the other patients and was in the habit of annoying them by sitting on their laps. She began to improve by the first week of August of the same year. She was discharged as cured on 3 September. She resided near the town. It was found on enquiry that she continued to be quite sane since the date of her discharge.

Mussumat Sonae, a Muslim, was admitted on 12 June. She was thirty-five years old. She was reported on the descriptive roll as 'wandering about' and abusive, as well as ill-treating people occasionally. The names of her relatives or her place of residence were not known. She had fits of violent excitement during which she was in the habit tearing off her clothes, exposing herself, and daubing her body with mud. At other times she alternatively danced or sang or screamed and rolled about on the ground. Her strength declined due to repeated paroxysms and she became more and more emaciated. She had diarrhoea for which she was given 'mistcrete' and tint opii (tincture of opium), and soup and sago for her diet. Diarrhoea could be controlled temporarily but she could not be cured and died on 13 December.

Mussumat Felly was admitted on 28 August at the age of twenty-seven. The descriptive roll did not register any information regarding her caste, place of residence, or relatives. This explained that she was not admitted by her family friends, but was probably picked up from the street by the chowkidars. Usually, under such circumstances it was not possible to know about a patient's previous case history. At the asylum, her insanity manifested itself in immoderate fits of singing and dancing. At times, she enquired about her son. She was occasionally violent and was confined twice to solitary cells for striking other patients. She worked at the dhenkee and cleaned cotton. Her menstruation was regular.

Mussumat Paneekhatee was admitted on 12 September. She was thirty-two years old. She belonged to the lower caste. She was sent from Kamroop where she had been found wandering in the jungles at night. Initially she was violent and was kept under restraint, afterwards she became quiet. At the time of her admission she continued to talk incoherently, indulged in immoderate fits of singing and dancing, but gradually became silent. She even tried to hide herself from observation. She was once put into solitary confinement for tearing her clothes. Paneekhatee was inclined towards work, and was quiet and well-behaved. She dressed properly and continued to amend daily.

Mussumat Hurmonee was admitted on 9 October. She was twenty years old, and was a prostitute. Hurmonee was sent from Furredpore. She was reported in the 'descriptive roll' as having been in a hospital at Furredpore for two months on account of syphilis, of which she had been cured. Based on her previous hospital record, she was diagnosed as an insane person. But at the time of admission at the Dacca Asylum, her mind was more settled. She showed no symptoms of insanity while she was in the asylum. Hurmonee was at first silent and averse to answering questions, but afterwards she stated that she had been out of her mind at Furreedpore. As she gradually improved the medical officers decided to discharge her on 8 December.

Mussumat Chunder Mony was admitted on 14 November at the age of thirty-five. She belonged to the Kayet caste and was a cultivator by profession. She was described in the records as an 'idiot' who was unable to do anything for herself. She was sent to the asylum from the district of Faridpur in Bangladesh. She was quiet and inoffensive, and was weak in her lower extremities. When any person approached her, she made a number of salaams, and touched the ground with her forehead.

Fyzun Meerasen, a Muslim, was readmitted on 25 May 1842. Fyzun's was a case of substance consumption. She was cured and discharged to the care of her sister on 22 May. Her addiction problem relapsed and within two days she was back to smoking ganja, and was readmitted. At the time of her admission she was very 'excited and unmanageable'. She rolled on the ground and was abusive. During her stay at the asylum she was also confined to the solitary cell for being physically violent towards one of the patients. She tore off her clothes and refused to work. In less than a month's time, the situation improved. Hence, she was employed at the asylum labour on 15 June and gradually showed signs of was rationality in her conversation. She even began her prayers regularly. She was finally discharged cured on 24 October. Therefore, 'excitement' and 'addiction' were the primary reasons for her mental illness and once that was cured the medical officers considered her suitable for release.

Aoduh, a Hindu, was admitted to the asylum on 20 October 1842, at the age of nineteen. No descriptive roll accompanied this patient and nothing was known of her previous history. During her admission at the asylum, she did not have clothes on her body. She was violent, she refused to eat, and tore off her clothes and blanket. She had high fever on 15 November. She also suffered from dysentery. Aoduh finally died on 29 November.[107]

The cases of Commulle, Noyanbee, and Airhollah were different not only because a post-mortem examination was done after their deaths, but also because the medical officers gave a detailed report regarding the condition of their brain, chest, and abdomen. These cases were complicated. This showed that by the 1860s, the definition of insanity was taking a complex turn. It was not enough to only describe the malady as 'derangement of the mind'; post mortem reports were written with special emphasis on brain, chest, and abdomen conditions.[108] This explained a gradual attempt to understand insanity as a disease, while also revealing the beginning of post-mortem examinations on the bodies of patients as sites of medical examinations and knowledge (see Table 3.7).

Commulle was admitted at the Dacca Asylum on 10 August 1861 at the age of thirty. She suffered from chronic mania at the time of admission. Whenever she was excited she used to set her house on fire, which proved risky to her family and to her neighbours. Her insanity was first diagnosed by a physician from outside the asylum on the basis of the neighbours' and family's reports. On her admission, the medical officers concluded that her poor financial condition due to 'loss of money' was the reason for her insanity. Commulle was at times extremely violent, and was diagnosed with homicidal tendencies. She was also 'abusive, intractable, and irascible'. A year after her admission, she suffered from choleric diarrhoea on 14 April 1862. She died of this disease on 16 April 1862.[109] The post-mortem report stated that her heart and lungs were congested, and choleric bile was found in her abdomen.[110]

---

[107] Medical Board Proceedings, Number 18, April 1843, Enclosure to a Letter submitted by J. Tayler, Civil Surgeon, Dacca to Robert Brown, Superintending Surgeon, Dacca, 13 April 1843, NAI.

[108] For an understanding of post-mortem, see Mark Harrison, 'Morbid Anatomy in British India, 1770–1850', in *The Social History of Health and Medicine in Colonial India*, edited by Biswamoy Pati and Mark Harrison (Oxford: Routledge, 2009), 173–94.

[109] A. Simpson, 'Report on the Dacca Lunatic Asylum for the Year 1862,' *Annual Report on the Insane Asylums of Bengal for the Year 1862*.

[110] A. Simpson, 'Report on the Dacca Lunatic Asylum for the Year 1862,' *Annual Report on the Insane Asylums of Bengal for the Year 1862*.

Table 3.7 Casualty List, History, and Post-mortem Appearances of Three Female Inmates at the Dacca Lunatic Asylum in 1862

Name, Date of Admission, Age	Case History	Cause of Death	Brain	Chest	Abdomen
Commulle (female). Admitted from Dacca, 10 August 1861. Aetat 30. Mania Chronic	Cause of insanity assigned to loss of money; subjected at times to violent restraint, when excited said to have tendency to set fire to her house and to be dangerous to her neighbours, has homicidal tendencies; abusive, intractable, and irascible. Was attacked with choleric diarrhoea on 14 April 1862, and died in collapse	Choleraic diarrhoea, 16 April 1862	Body in good condition. Extremities collapsed. Membranes healthy. Slight venous congestion. No unusual serosity. Cortical and medullar substance healthy. Ventricles of normal size.	Lungs congested. Heart healthy. Fibrinous clot on both sides. Blood black.	Liver fatty. Gall bladder distended with green bile. Stomach full of watery fluid. Duodenum contained yellowish fluid. Ileum congested in large patches. Contents choleric fluid. Colon healthy. Contents a light colour thin pultaceous fluid of lumbrici in small intestines.

(Cont'd)

Table 3.7 (Contd)

Name, Date of Admission, Age	Case History	Cause of Death	Brain	Chest	Abdomen
Noyanbee (female). Admitted from Dacca, 12 March 1854. Aetat 40. Mania Chronic.	No previous history obtained. On admission subject to paroxysms of violence at long intervals; imbecile, sleeps, reserved, temper good, intractable, incoherent, and restless. Has goitre. In June 1861 became addicted to drinking her urine: blistered over the labia which prevented her from doing so anymore. Was seized with cholera on 2 June 1862 which proceeded to collapse, partial reaction ensued, and she died in a state of exhaustion.	Cholera in collapse, 7 June 1862	Venous congestion. No unusual quantity of serum under membranes. Ventricles small.	Lungs healthy, congested posteriorly. Heart healthy. Blood black and watery. Fibrinous clots in large vessels.	Liver healthy. Gall bladder distended. Small intestines congested in patches. No Lumbrici. Colon healthy. Kidney healthy.

| Airhollah (female). Admitted from Dacca, 12 November 1859. Aetat 35. Mania Choric | Stated in Descriptive Roll to be abusive and violent. Sent in by the police. On admission imbecile, sleepless, intractable, irascible, incoherent, melancholic, uproarious, and talkative. From February 1861, health declined, and she became cachectic, scratching and picking the skin off her legs and arms. In January 1862, pinches herself, takes off pieces of her skin and eats it, and sucks her blood. Suffered with fever and diarrhoea, and gradually sunk into a state of extreme anaemia, and ultimately died from a slight attack of diarrhoea. | Extreme anaemia, diarrhoea and fever, 2 December 1862 | Membranes healthy. Slight serous effusion on surface, and into ventricles on extremity. Anaemic. Condition of the brain otherwise healthy. | Lungs healthy. Heart slight effusion into pericardium. Muscular structure of right ventricle very fatty. | Liver extreme fatty degeneration. Colon light clay, almost white. Gall bladder distended. Intestines anaemic. Contents fluid foeculence with little or no bile. No ulceration of colon. |

Source: A. Simpson, 'Report on the Dacca Lunatic Asylum for the Year 1862,' *Annual Reports and Returns of the Insane Asylums in Bengal for the Year 1862*, compiled by J. McClelland, Officiating Principal Inspector General, Medical Department (Calcutta: Military Orphan Press, 1863), NAI.

Noyanbee was admitted at the Dacca Asylum on 12 March 1854 at the age of forty. No previous history was obtained. After her admission she would have paroxysms of violence at long intervals. Her temperament was good. Other symptoms of her insanity included: 'imbecility, reserve, intractability, incoherence, and restlessness', although her death on 7 June 1862 was due to cholera and not the symptoms from which she suffered. She also had goitre. By June 1861, the asylum physicians noticed that she was addicted to drinking her urine. According to the physicians, she could not continue it for long because she got blisters on her labia, which caused irritation. By June 1862, she had cholera, and finally died of exhaustion. The post-mortem report stated that her brain and lungs were congested but her liver was found healthy.[111] Physicians outside the asylums also recognized symptoms of mental illness as did the asylum physicians. While the doctors, either inside or outside the asylum, could detect symptoms of insanity as understood during the time, none were specialized in its treatment. It also showed that insanity was yet to be wholly considered as a mental disease, which needed specialized treatment.

Airhollah was admitted at the Dacca Asylum on 12 November 1859 at the age of thirty-five. She suffered from chronic mania. She was described as abusive and violent on the descriptive roll. She was sent to the asylum by the police. On admission she was 'imbecile, sleepless, intractable, irascible, incoherent, melancholic, uproarious, and talkative'. From February 1861, her health declined, and she became cachectic, scratching and picking the skin off her legs and arms. In January 1862 she began pinching herself and took off pieces of her skin and ate them, and also sucked her own blood. She suffered due to fever and diarrhoea, and gradually sank into a state of extreme anaemia, and ultimately died from a slight attack of diarrhoea.[112] The post-mortem report showed her brain and lungs to be healthy but her abdomen showed signs of anaemia.[113]

---

[111] A. Simpson, 'Report on the Dacca Lunatic Asylum for the Year 1862,' *Annual Report on the Insane Asylums of Bengal for the Year 1862.*

[112] A. Simpson, 'Report on the Dacca Lunatic Asylum for the Year 1862,' *Annual Report on the Insane Asylums of Bengal for the Year 1862.*

[113] A. Simpson, 'Report on the Dacca Lunatic Asylum for the Year 1862,' *Annual Report on the Insane Asylums of Bengal for the Year 1862.*

Mussumat Shonah was admitted at the Cuttack Lunatic Asylum on April 1867, while suffering from monomania. She did not complain of any sickness, and took her food on time. On one morning of July 1869, the medical officers observed that her legs from the feet upwards had become oedematous, and she died suddenly at noon on the same day. Post-mortem examination was done within three hours of her death. According to the officer, the brain appeared healthy, the pericardium was much distended with serum, and the lungs were congested; the remaining organs were healthy. She was a patient in the asylum for two years, three months, and twenty-five days.[114]

Joygoon was admitted at the Dacca Asylum from the district of Tipperah. She suffered from chronic dementia, and died in 1870 in the asylum. The causes of her illness as stated by the Asylum Visitor were mania and debility. Another woman, Borborah Khotany, admitted from Nowgong, suffered from acute mania, and also died in 1870. The reasons as stated by the medical officer were mania due to chronic meningitis, and chronic dysentery.[115]

At the Cuttack Lunatic Asylum in 1872, a woman, aged forty, was admitted for seven and a half years. She was under treatment for two months before her death due to chronic diarrhoea. She died on 1 March. Her disease was diagnosed as chronic mania. Another woman at the asylum, aged fifty-eight, was admitted for three years. For several months before her death, she suffered due to ill health. She had 'oedematous swelling of the limbs', and suffered from recurring attacks of dysentery, and died of debility. She was as a chronic mania patient.[116]

Another old woman suffering from ill health stayed in the asylum for eight years. She suffered from anaemia with 'dropsiacal swellings', and

[114] Letter sent to the Secretary Inspector General of Hospitals, Indian Medical Department, Calcutta, from Surgeon J. Macdonald Superintendent, Cuttack Lunatic Asylum, Cuttack, dated 12 January 1870, in *Annual Report on the Insane Asylums in Bengal for the Year 1869* by J. Murray, M.D, Inspector General of Hospitals, Indian Medical Department (Calcutta: Bengal Secretariat Office, 1870), NAI.

[115] Bengal Proceedings, Medical Department, Number 10, 1870, Visitor's Report on the Dacca Asylum, NAI.

[116] H. Cayley, 'Report on the Cuttack Lunatic Asylum for the Year 1872,' *Annual Report on the Insane Asylums of Bengal for the Year 1872.*

died on 22 October 1872. She suffered from melancholy. According to the Superintendent of the asylum, in cases of confirmed melancholia and chronic dementia, the general health after a time almost began to fail. He further justified the cause of death thus:

> In a small asylum where the numbers were not sufficient to keep up a steady average, an excessive mortality in one year, and a very low rate in another, was often mere accidental circumstances.[117]

In 1872, at the Moydapore Lunatic Asylum, a woman was admitted on charges of murder. On her admission the superintendent found her quite sane. She later stated that her desire in life was to commit suicide and to take her child with her in the next birth. Therefore, she killed the child, and before she could do the same to herself, she was seized and prevented. It was assumed that either the family or the neighbours intervened to stop her. This case was different in that while the Civil Surgeon did not diagnose her as insane, the Judge considered her 'mad' and sent her to the asylum for treatment. This was a case of medical jurisprudence, where medically she was considered mentally fit, but by legal measures she was considered unfit. The Civil Surgeon finally recommended her release.[118]

DELIVERY IN THE ASYLUM

There were some instances of women giving birth in the asylum. While such instances were often reported at the European Lunatic Asylum, it was not so common in 'native' asylums. By the late nineteenth century, the replacement of *mehtarnee*s (female sweepers) by *dhai*s (midwives) at the 'native' asylums of Bengal[119] proved that instances of women were giving birth, gradually increased, although there was no further discussion on this.

[117] H. Cayley, 'Report on the Cuttack Lunatic Asylum for the Year 1872,' *Annual Report on the Insane Asylums of Bengal for the Year 1872*.

[118] J. M. Coates, 'Report on the Moydapore Lunatic Asylum for the Year 1872,' *Annual Report on the Insane Asylums of Bengal for the Year 1872*.

[119] Municipal Department, Medical Branch, Number 15, February 1900, Copy of Remarks made by Surgeon T. H. Hendeley Inspector General of Civil Hospitals on his visit to the Dacca Lunatic Asylum, dated 26 July 1898, APAC, BL.

The superintendent of an asylum not only decided the symptoms and causes of insanity, but also the fate of the insane in case she delivered a child or already had a child. In such a situation, it was the superintendent who decided whether the child should stay with the mother or not. The case of Mrs Butler exemplified this. Mrs Butler delivered a child in January 1839, in Beardsmore's private asylum. She had already borne a child prior to her admission at the asylum. Because she was in a state of 'fury', he recommended to the Medical Board that the child be removed to the Orphan School. According to the superintendent of the asylum,

> the mother's state of mind being such, as to render the separation of her infant from her a measure of absolute necessity, in consequent of the frequent paroxysms of fury, to which she is subject and as she appears quiet indifferent about this infant, and does not afford it nourishment.[120]

In another instance, Mrs Gunnan's infant son was also sent to the Orphan School of Calcutta.[121] This showed that all children of female inmates of the Bhawanipore Lunatic Asylum were sent to the Orphan School. Unfortunately, in the course of time when those women were sent back to England, their children continued to stay in the Orphan School in Calcutta.

Esquirol's understanding of insanity was divided into physical and moral causes, of which menstrual disorder was one of the physical causes of insanity. The disorder and cessation of menses were important reasons for such mental illnesses. He further stated that moral causes gave rise to dementia more frequently among women than among men. According to Pinel, sudden joy and sudden grief also produced dementia.[122]

In March 1857, Mrs Anne Eliza Hoyle was confined in the Bhawanipore Lunatic Asylum in Calcutta. Almost after ten years, in 1868, her daughter, Mrs Mary Beck wrote a letter to the Medical Board,

[120] Medical Board Proceedings, 7 January 1839, Enclosure Attached to a Letter sent to Adam Smith, Member of the Medical Board and also Visiting Member of the Bhawanipore Lunatic Asylum for the month of January 1839 by J. Bearsdmore, dated 2 February 1839, NAI.

[121] Medical Board Proceedings, 7 January 1839, Enclosure Attached to a Letter sent to from J. Beardsmore to Adam Smith.

[122] Daniel Tuke, 'On the Various Forms of Mental Disorder', edited by John Charles Bucknill, *Asylum Journal*, 3 (1856–7): 88, WL.

stating that she and her other siblings were 'anxious' to know about their mother's recovery. On her enquiry at the European Lunatic Asylum, the Superintendent could not give any further detail regarding Mrs Anne Eliza Hoyle. At a much later stage she got to know that her mother had been transferred to an asylum in England. Following this, Mrs Anne's daughter wrote to the Bethlehem Hospital in London and enquired if the superintendent of that institution had any information about her mother. In reply she got to know that they did not. She was informed by an individual who had seen her before she left the country that her mother was quite reasonable in all her conservation, and that she also made enquiries about her children. Anxiously stating these helpless circumstances, the daughter of Mrs Anne implored the Secretary to the State to enquire into the matter in order to find out which asylum she was sent back to in England. She also expressed her wish to write to the Governor General for further clarifications.[123] The Secretary of State replied that he would try and help her and inform her on receiving any information.[124] As there was no further discussion on the issue, it was difficult to find out what happened to Hoyle and whether she finally managed to unite with her family; such was the fate of the insane who were abandoned by their family members or who had no one else to look after them.

Different types of medicines administered to inmates primarily included tonics, sedatives, and purgatives. Sedatives were given to control signs of excitement, to make the patient sleep. Purgatives were administered to restore the normal movement of bowels. For improving their state of debility, dosages of tonics were given. It was not 'feminizing madness' in totality, rather there was an emerging trend that perceived 'male insanity' as separate from women's. This understanding of male insanity as different from women's insanity was not only determined by the biological differences between both the sexes, but also the socially-constructed difference, which understood woman's normality

[123] Home Department, Public Proceedings, 11 July 1868, Letter sent to E. C. Bayley, Secretary to the Government of India, Simla from Mrs Mary Beck, Daughter of the Patient, dated 16 May 1868, NAI.

[124] Home Department, Public Proceedings, 11 July 1868, Letter sent to E. C. Bayley, NAI, Letter sent from G. Geoghegan, Under Secretary to the Government of India to Mrs M. Beck, Delhi Railway Contractor's Office, Meerut, Number 2882, Simla, dated 8 July 1868, NAI.

and abnormality in terms of their menstrual cycle, her weak physical constitution, and her emotional exuberances.

Women hardly had any place to return to on being discharged. *Abalabandhab*, a Bengali newspaper, in 1873, stated that the custom among the 'natives' of Bengal was to refuse to accept an imprisoned woman who returned to the house or into her circle of friends. It further stated that a man—even if guilty of the most heinous crime against religion, mortality, or society, and even if he had been condemned to a period to imprisonment—immediately upon his release, was welcomed back by his family and to the circle of his friends, and 'no one turned towards him a dark look or spoke a word of reproach'. But if a woman was found guilty of any crime, or sentenced to imprisonment simply because she could not offer satisfactory proof of her innocence, she had no place to return to. An unmarried woman sent to prison could never be married and a married woman was immediately abandoned, and her husband would marry another. A widow was never received back by any of her own or her husband's friends. A woman, therefore, released from a prison had nowhere to go. Her only place of refuge under such circumstances became a brothel.[125] This probably held true of asylum inmates as well, which often became their last resort even after they were cured.

Unlike England, where as Elaine Showalter had pointed out, insanity could be defined as a 'female malady', the same was not applicable in case of India or Bengal. In Bengal, both men and women were admitted in the asylums. Although the number of women was lower than that of men, it did not by any means determine that women alone suffered from mental illnesses. Therefore, there was no 'feminizing of madness', but there was certainly a gendered definition of madness which was the result of both biological differences and the outcome of an imagined psycho-social factor, which viewed women as unsettled and prone to emotional exuberances, and therefore, prone to insanity. In this context, it is necessary to remember that as human beings, men are as emotional as women.

[125] *Abalabandhab*, Report on the Native Newspaper Report of Bengal, May 1873, NAI.

4

THE ROLE OF ASYLUM STAFF
IN THE TREATMENT OF INSANITY

ASYLUM STAFF MEMBERS WERE RESPONSIBLE for the treatment of the insane. They were to give them medicines, supervise their work, and oversee patients even when they were put in solitary confinement. Therefore, the establishment of the asylum staff was an indispensable constituent of the asylum management because they were responsible for the well-being, care, and management of the inmates in both European and 'native' asylums in the Lower Provinces of Bengal. The responsibility of the establishment was to intervene in the patient's daily life and regularize it in order to bring the patient back to a regular and 'normal' life. The asylum staff consisted of a 'native' doctor, and both European and 'native' Overseers. Depending on their composition, the duties of the asylum staff can be divided into two broad categories: the care staff and the maintenance staff. Although this distinction was clear-cut, their duties often overlapped. For instance, the *jemadar* (sweeper), *bheesty* (water-carrier) and peon not only took physical care of inmates, but were often posted as guards in the absence of *daroga*s (constables). They cleaned the compound and the cells, and fetched water for the asylum.

The care staff consisted of attendants, also known as keepers. The maintenance staff consisted of daroga, bheesty, jemadar, *mehtar* (sweeper), *mehtarnee* (female sweeper), *negaban* (attendant), *barkandaze* (an armed policeman), *dhobi* (washerman), *guala* (water carrier), *harkara* (conveyor of news), *mali* (gardener), cook, and tailor.

The establishment of the European Lunatic Asylum mainly included European and 'native' attendants, both male and female, one European Overseer, and a cook, guard, tailor, and gardener. The establishment of the European Lunatic Asylum was different from that of 'native' asylums; the total number of staff appointed in case of the former was always lower than in the latter. This was mainly because of two reasons; first, patients in the former asylum were divided into three classes: upper division, middle class and pauper 'lunatics'. Second, patients were only temporarily admitted in the European Lunatic Asylum; after a short duration of stay they were usually sent back to England for further treatment. During their journey to England, they were accompanied by European and 'native' attendants who, on completion of their duty, returned to the asylum. Although for these two reasons the maintenance costs of the establishment were higher in the European Asylum than in the latter, there was still another reason for the higher salary. This was because European, Eurasian and Anglo-Indian inmates[1] at the European Lunatic Asylum were maintained either by their family, friends, or relatives or by the government. But in the native asylums, patients were usually maintained by government funds. The number of patients admitted in each of the 'native' lunatic asylums was always higher than those admitted in the European Lunatic Asylum. European patients hardly had to do any work in the asylum whereas inmates in the 'native' asylums were involved in different laborious activities, which involved the supervision of more asylum staff. The profit gained from the labour of lunatics was often used to pay the asylum staff over and above their fixed payment from the government fund.

By the middle of the nineteenth century, with the growing debate on the replacement of mechanical restraint with non-mechanical restraint or moral treatment in England, there was an attempt by the asylum officials to shift the method of treatment of insanity from

---

[1] Although non-European patients like those stated here were treated at the European Lunatic Asylum, those who did not have any relatives, friends, or family in England or Calcutta to take care of them were eventually sent to the 'native' asylums of Bengal for further treatment.

mechanical to the moral. The most notable proponents of moral treatment amongst many others were Daniel Tuke, an English physician (1827–1895), and John Conolly, an English physician (1794–1866). Their works on moral treatment were practised in various asylums in England and also taught in the medical schools there. The members of the Medical Board, the European asylum doctors, and superintendents who practised in the asylums of India were educated in the medical colleges of Edinburgh and England. Therefore, on their appointment in charge of the asylums of Bengal, they implemented their medical training in practice. Although the asylum staff was already appointed in India from early nineteenth century, this study establishes how over time their role changed and became more significant. The reason is that it was through the asylum staff that the moral treatment of insanity was practised in the asylums of Bengal. For instance, instead of putting the patients into handcuffs, waistcoats, straitjackets, and so on, the asylum staff was employed to take care of them. According to Daniel Tuke, the practice of non-restraint was complemented by 'superior power of the attendants', although 'manual detention by holding the hands of the lunatics' was allowed to some extent.[2] Under this new method of treatment, the asylum staff were perceived by European doctors as friends, companions, and guardians of patients. It was through them that the proponents of moral treatment of insanity controlled and changed the way mental illness was understood and treated in the asylums. Therefore, it is important to study this establishment to know their social composition, the rules and regulations set for them, and to see how far their presence changed the mode of treatment practised in the asylums.

COMPOSITION OF THE ESTABLISHMENT

Good conduct and a sense of responsibility along with gentleness and a caring attitude towards the patients were the necessary criteria for appointments in the post-asylum staff. They were also selected on the

---

[2] Daniel Tuke, *Moral Management of the Insane and the Various Contrivances which Have Been Adopted Instead of Mechanical Restraint* (London: John Churchill, 1854), 109, WL.

basis of their intelligence and smartness.[3] Andrew Scull, in his discussions on asylums of England, pointed out that the attendants were recruited from

> the unemployed of other professions … if they possess physical strength and of tolerable reputation for sobriety, it is enough; and the latter quality is frequently dispensed with. They enter upon their duties completely ignorant of what insanity is.[4]

While this was the necessary criteria for the post of the care staff, a strong physique was an added criterion for the post of an attendant. Although the idea was to replace mechanical restraint with the care of attendants, this particular necessity explained that mechanical coercion was only replaced by physical coercion. As Daniel Tuke further pointed out, 'much conflict between attendant and patient will be saved when the latter is conscious of the entire hopelessness of the result of any trial of strength'.[5]

The asylum staff was an indispensable part of the asylum management. Therefore, whenever any plan for a new asylum was proposed by the administration officials, the composition and the number of asylum staff was also decided along with it. The total size of the staff varied from one asylum to another. For instance, the size of the asylum staff proposed along with the plan for the establishment of the Insane Hospital of Calcutta in 1804, included a jemadar, two cooks, eight peons, two matrons, and two bheesties,[6] whereas the staff proposed along with the proposal for the establishment of the Dacca Asylum in 1805 included one native doctor, four peons, two cooks, two mehters, and two bheesties.[7]

---

[3] Home, Public, Medical, Number 11, December 1871, Letter sent to the Deputy Inspector General of Hospitals, Dacca Circle, from Dr Wise, NAI.

[4] Andrew Scull, *The Most Solitary of Afflictions: Madness and Society in Britain 1700–1900* (New Haven and London: Yale University Press, 1993), 173.

[5] Tuke, *Moral Management of the Insane*, 101, WL.

[6] Judicial Department, Criminal Branch Proceedings, Numbers 17–20, 1804, Letter sent by George Dowdeswell, Secretary to the Government of Bengal, Calcutta, Police Office, dated 5 August 1804, WBSA.

[7] Judicial Department, Criminal Branch Proceedings, Number 7, 1805, Letter sent to G. Dowdeswell, Secretary to the Government in the Judicial Department from W. Parket, Magistrate of Dacca, dated 19 March 1805, WBSA.

Certain factors determined the size and composition of asylum staff. First, there was the location of the asylum—whether it was built at the centre of the town or in a remote place far away from the central location. For instance, according to A. Fleming, because the Moydapore Asylum was located at a distance from the central locality—almost four to five miles away from Berhampore—it was difficult to appoint staff at that asylum. None were willing to join the service as they got better employment elsewhere. Those who were employed also resigned eventually. As a result, the post of the Hindu cook remained vacant. Food for the Hindu patients was prepared by one of the Hindu inmates.[8]

Second, the size of the asylum building—the total area covered, the number of rooms and wards, and the number of inmates—was a deciding factor for the space allotted to the resident asylum staff. During the early nineteenth century, when there were very few asylums in Bengal and the number of 'lunatics' admitted was also low, the asylum staff was recruited in proportion to this. This situation not only changed over the century, but also got complicated as more asylums were established and more patients were admitted to them. Gradually, a new problem emerged while recruiting them, which was the issue of their pay. It had put the management of the asylum in a state of crisis. Several factors related to it made the position of the asylum staff difficult. For instance, by the 1870s at the Dacca Asylum, when there were instances of theft, attendants were accused. According to the medical officers, they were engaged in such activities due to their low pay scale. In order to control the situation, guards were appointed to monitor the activities of the attendants.[9] This shows that the asylum staff was not only recruited to care for and maintain the inmates, but also to inspect each other's activities. The size of the asylum staff, therefore, differed from one asylum to another.

The availability and the preference of staff was another reason why their number and composition varied. The staff recruited for asylum jobs

[8] A. Fleming, 'Report on the Moorshedabad Lunatic Asylum for the Year 1862,' NAI.

[9] Home, Public, Medical, Number 11, Letter from Dr Wise to Deputy Inspector General of Hospitals.

were not specially trained for the purpose. They were a group of people who were not expected to be educated, but had to be of good physique and moral character. This class was mainly recruited for menial jobs. Hence, they were also recruited in various institutions, other than in asylums. Initially the asylum staff was recruited from the locality which mainly comprised. But over time, 'up-country' men were preferred. For instance, men who had served in various capacities under an Overseer in the horse artillery in their former years were appointed. Some of them were Punjabis who, after their discharge from regiments, had settled in the neighbourhoods of Calcutta. Content with their service at the asylum, they also asked their fellow countrymen residing outside Bengal to join the post of the asylum staff.[10] The class composition gradually changed as more non-Bengalis were recruited but their duties remained the same.

With the increase in the number of asylums, jails, and administrative offices, the demand for local men for such posts also increased. The low pay scale in the asylums, in comparison to other institutions, made them look for opportunities elsewhere. In this context the Superintendent of the Dacca Lunatic Asylum stated that the inadequate pay drew the 'worst' Bengalis for the post. According to him, a Bengali attendant under such circumstances took no interest in his work, and having little to gain, he accepted the post with hesitation, and received a dismissal salary without regret.[11]

The medical officials were doubtful about the duties of the 'native' asylum staff. They mostly considered them as untrustworthy and misfits in their job. For instance, regarding the treatment of 'native' attendants towards the Europeans, John Bucknill stated that

> there exists a peculiar condition well deserving of notice. That is, the sense of humiliation or degradation, which certain classes, soldiers and sailors in particular, are in the habit of attaching coercion by the hands

[10] A. Payne, 'Report on the Dullunda Lunatic Asylum for the Year 1869,' sent to the Deputy Inspector General of Hospitals, Presidency Circle, Fort William, Dullunda, dated 1 January 1870, in *Annual Report on the Insane Asylums in Bengal for the Year 1869* by J. Murray, Inspector General of Hospitals, Indian Medical Department (Calcutta: Bengal Secretariat Office 1870), NAI.

[11] Home, Public, Medical, Number 11, Letter from Dr Wise to Deputy Inspector General of Hospitals.

of native attendants. In asylums in India, restraint ought to be applied exclusively by European attendants where their service cannot be had things supply the next best instrumentality, because they are likely to cause less resistance, and to leave no impression of humiliation, whereas coercion by the hands of natives is almost certain of producing both effects.[12]

Similar views were also expressed by the Civil Surgeon of Moorshedabad regarding the 'native' attendants employed at the 'native' asylum. According to him, 'Natives are utterly untrustworthy, and have no sympathy with their unfortunate fellow countrymen suffering from various forms of insanity.'[13]

Other than the care and maintenance staff, the role of 'native' doctor and both 'native' and European Overseers are also significant. The native doctor was trained in Western medicine, and usually resided in the quarters within the asylum. Overseers, who also resided within the compound of the asylum, were mainly appointed to look after the overall maintenance of the asylum staff including the native doctor. The asylum staff worked under the supervision of the Overseer, who was expected to be a good natured and equable person. He did not have to possess any specific skill for the post. Therefore, amongst the entire staff, the 'native' doctor was the only educated and medically trained person.

DUTIES OF THE ESTABLISHMENT

The medical officers were dependent on the asylum staff for their regular reports on the inmates. A medical officer often gathered information from the asylum staff on his visits to the asylum. During one such visit,

[12] John Charles Bucknill, 'Report on East Indian Asylums,' in *The Asylum Journal of Mental Sciences*, Volume 5, edited by John Charles Bucknill, 1858–59, WL.

[13] Home, Public Proceedings, Medical, Bengal, Number 42, 14 May 1860, Enclosure of a letter from D. J. A. Guise, Civil Surgeon of Moorshedabad to F. Anderson, Superintending Surgeon Barrackpore, Number 65, dated 25 October 1859, Enclosed in the letter from T. Cantor, Superintendent of the Asylums at Bhawanipore and Dullunda to the Secretary to the Director General of the Medical Department, letter number 142, dated 24 October 1859, APAC, BL.

in 1821, to the European Lunatic Asylum, one of the members of the Medical Board wrote that the questions asked to the staff on duty

> were purely of an ordinary nature and which however necessary that we should be informed regarding them, could not in our judgement be liable to misconception as they assuredly were not meant to trench upon the privileges of the Surgeon. They were such as we deemed it to be our doubted right as vested with the general control and superintendence of the house to put and which consistently with the due performance of our duty we were strictly bound to put.[14]

Based on the report of the staff, the Board not only decided upon the course of treatment for the lunatics, but also decided about patients of the European Asylum who were sent to England for further treatment.

Other than their duty as informers, they were engaged in various daily activities. One was giving medicines as prescribed by doctors. But, it was attendants who had no medical qualifications, who were put in charge of such a delicate job. Under such circumstances, one cannot be sure of the medicines they gave and whether they gave the right dosage to the patients. Another difficult situation arose during emergencies. As they were in constant contact with inmates rather than the doctors, during emergencies they were the first to deal with the patient. The doctors were available only when the attendants informed them about such a situation. Therefore, it was the attendant who took the decision about the patient's illness and administered the medicine; they called for the doctor only if they thought it was necessary. This involved an important medico-ethical issue. Attendants gradually acquired the role of deciding the fate of patients instead of the doctors. This made the treatment of inmates difficult. 'Lunacy' needed specialized treatment, and how far the attendants were capable of doing that was doubtful. In 1869 at Dullunda, three cases of illness were brought to the notice of the medical officials by the attendants.[15] The role played by them added a new dimension to their work. Attendants were also employed

[14] Medical Board Proceedings, Number 21, 19 February 1821, Letter sent to Colonel Casement, Secretary to Government in the Military Department by Members of the Medical Board, dated 17 February 1821, NAI.

[15] Medical Board Proceedings, Number 21, Letter from Members of the Medical Board to Colonel Casement, 17 February 1821.

in 'spontaneously' looking for illnesses among the inhabitants of the place, and without this search,[16] according to the superintendent of the asylum, the illnesses often progressed unnoticed. The usual practice was to keep up an unremitting search for illnesses throughout the day, which did not end even when his day's work was over, or when the surgeon's visit was over. This practice was dangerous, because the attendants were not medically trained. Therefore, at a time when the definition of insanity itself was in the making, the views of medically untrained persons on the treatment of insanity were very problematic. The practitioners of moral treatment were against the medical treatment of insanity, which they often considered as extremely harmful for the recovery of a patient. According to John Conolly, the medical officers were 'ill educated men of illiberal views, and 'opposed to every improvement'.[17] Therefore, it was evident why the medical qualifications of attendants could never be an essential requisite for managing the insane.

In 1836, the Officiating Secretary of the Medical Board on his visit to the European Lunatic Asylum stated that

the attendants have appeared to be capriciously changed, and their numbers increased or diminished without regard to the wants of the inmates. A sufficiency of male and female keepers, not hired by the day or week like common labourers, but permanently engaged and taught by experience and appropriate instruction to manage persons suffering under the various forms of mental derangement, is in our humble opinion indispensable to an institution worthy of the patronage of Government.[18]

Therefore, it was expected that the position of the asylum staff was a permanent one and the medical officers in charge of them were supposed to train them in their duties.

[16] Medical Board Proceedings, Number 21, Letter from Members of the Medical Board to Colonel Casement, 17 February 1821.

[17] John Charles Bucknill, Review of *The Treatment of the Insane without Mechanical Restraint*, by John Conolly, *Asylum Journal* 3 (1856–57): 256, WL.

[18] Letter sent to Jameson, Secretary to the Medical Board, from James Ranken, Officiating Secretary Medical Board, dated 7 May 1836 in Correspondence of the Medical Board in *The Quarterly Journal of the Calcutta Medical and Physical Society*, 1 October 1837, WL.

According to Charles Mercier, the duties of attendants were of the most responsible character, because a brief lapse in vigilance or attention often resulted in catastrophes, like the injury or death of inmates under their care that often led to a disaster to their own careers.[19] He further stated that the role of the attendants could be divided into the care of the insane and the treatment that revolved around it. While the former consisted of care for their safety, cleanliness, comfort, and welfare, the latter involved cure of their mental and bodily disorders.[20]

At the Dacca Lunatic Asylum the jemadar inspected the clothes and blankets of the inmates and occasionally changed them as well. The attendants in charge fed the inmates two meals in a day, once at 8 AM and then again at 3 PM. The attendants were also responsible for supplying the inmates with the daily allowance of tobacco, betel nut, and occasionally, fruits. These was mainly given to the patients as incentives, and attendants had full control over its distribution. It was the attendants' task to put the blankets outside every morning on a bamboo framework erected for the purpose. The clothes of all the patients were washed once a week. The wards were washed out and fumigated every morning and once a week the floors, doors, windows, and walls of the several rooms were cleaned. The walls were also whitewashed by attendants wherever necessary.[21] Although it was the attendants' duty to clean the cells, wards, and verandas, the medical officers expected the inmates to perform similar duties as well.

At the Patna Lunatic Asylum, the attendants' duty was to clean drains regularly and whitewash the asylum quarterly. The aim was to keep the building airy for the comfort of the patients.[22] Along with the asylum staff, inmates participated equally in similar as a part of their labour

---

[19] Charles Mercier, *The Attendants Companion: A Manual of the Duties of Attendants in Lunatic Asylums* (London: J. & A. Churchill, 1898), 1, WL.

[20] Mercier, *The Attendants Companion*, 4.

[21] Medical Board Proceedings, May 1842, Letter sent to Officiating Superintending Surgeon Robert Brown from J. Taylor, Civil Surgeon, Dacca, dated 2 May 1842, NAI.

[22] Medical Board Proceedings, May 1842, Letter sent to J. Marshall, Superintending Surgeon, Dinapore from Civil Surgeon Samuel Davies, Patna Civil Surgeon's Office, dated 2 May 1842, NAI.

therapy, which was exacted by the medical officials on the pretext of their treatment. For instance, when the floors of the asylum at Russapaglah were found damp, patients constructed raised platforms or *machan*s of bamboo to make their own beds.[23]

In 1842, A. Kean stated that the establishment staff of the asylum gave 'little trouble' and the 'native' doctor was diligent and attentive.[24] The principal aim of management, according to the Civil Surgeon, was to treat the inmates with kindness, and to encourage employment and self-disciplining. Patients who managed to elude the vigilance of the keeper were punished.[25] This was usually done by putting them in solitary confinement. In the absence of the medical officer, the attendants were also in charge of monitoring punishments.

At times when there was a scarcity of asylum staff due to their low pay scale, the medical officers employed prison convicts as staff members of the asylum. This engagement, therefore, blurred the dividing line between the convict of a jail and the non-criminal asylum staff, thereby creating a homogeneous group across two different places of confinement. Also, it provided the space for a free mixing between the prisoners in jail and the inmates. At the Dacca Lunatic Asylum, where the asylum and the jail were situated next to each other, convicts of the Dacca Jail were appointed in the asylum as mehtars, and dhobis at the cost of Rs 4 per month.[26] Later, by 1862, under orders of the Lieutenant Governor, convict sweepers of the asylum were discontinued because it became difficult to maintain them at lower rates. With the sanction of Rs 6 for each sweeper as per the revised rules for 'native'

[23] Medical Board Proceedings, Number 9, 30 September 1847, Letter sent to John Forsyth, Secretary to Medical Board from Dr Lamb, Officiating Superintending Surgeon, Presidency, NAI.

[24] Medical Board Proceedings, May 1842, Letter sent to W. Findon, Superintending Surgeon Presidency Division from A. Kean, Civil Assistant Surgeon, Moorshedabad, dated 25 April 1842, NAI.

[25] Medical Board Proceedings, May 1842, Letter from A. Kean, Civil Assistant Surgeon, Moorshedabad, dated 15 September 1841, NAI.

[26] Home, Public Proceedings, Medical, Bengal, Number 11, 23 August 1862, Letter sent to W. Thomson, Deputy Inspector General of Hospitals from A. Simpson, Superintendent Lunatic Asylum, Dacca, dated 25 February 1862, APAC, BL.

lunatic asylums, the convicted sweepers were once again recruited. Rational criminal patients were also employed in the asylum labour. They usually assisted the attendants in serving meals for inmates, and preserving order and regularity.[27]

By 1862, at the weekly distribution of clean clothes, the inmates were called by their numbers and clothes were distributed. Attendants were held responsible for any missing cloth, unless they were torn in which case, they were brought to the Overseer for mending. One of the keepers was particularly appointed for the bathing duties.[28] In order to maintain hygiene and cleanliness of the toilets and cells, the dry earth conservancy system was introduced into the asylum by Dr Beatson in 1865. The entire burden of night soil was carried outside the asylum in iron carts by the attendants.[29] But by 1870, the situation changed. Toilets covered with boxes full of dry earth were constructed and mehtars were appointed to go around the wards several times at night to throw dry earth into the pans. Dry earth was also strewn on the floors of those patients who were thought to have filthy habits. During the day time, patients used the garden are, which was also covered with dry earth by the mehtars, for the same purpose. The sewage of the asylum, after it was deodorized, was buried in pits in the garden outside the boundary wall by the mehtars. As one patch of ground became exhausted, it was tilled, and another place was appropriated for burying the sewage.[30]

The role of barkandazes was significant. They not only took care of inmates after admission but were also responsible for their safe journey to the asylum. For instance, they were responsible for the care and 'kind treatment' of patients on the road before they were admitted to the asylum

[27] A. Simpson, 'Report on the Dacca Lunatic Asylum for the Year 1862,' sent to W. Thomson, Deputy Inspector General of Hospitals, Dacca, *Annual Reports and Returns of the Insane Asylums in Bengal for the Years 1862–66* by J. McClleland, NAI.

[28] A. Simpson, 'Report on the Dacca Lunatic Asylum for the Year 1862,' *Annual Reports and Returns of the Insane Asylums in Bengal for the Years 1862–66.*

[29] A. Simpson, 'Report on the Dacca Lunatic Asylum for the Year 1862,' *Annual Reports and Returns of the Insane Asylums in Bengal for the Years 1862–66.*

[30] James Wise, 'Report on the Dacca Lunatic Asylum,' *Annual Report on the Insane Asylums in Bengal for the Year 1871*, J. Campbell Brown, NAI.

in the presence of the Magistrate or the Civil Surgeon.[31] They were also in charge of settling quarrels and fights amongst the patients. In 1869, at the Dacca Lunatic Asylum, there was a fight between two male inmates. The barkandaze pursued and seized one, and brought him before a jemadar, who was in charge of the patients. This was reported to the Overseer, who at once attended to the injured inmate and sent him to the hospital.[32]

While they were to control such outbreaks amongst the patients, they were also actually to blame for creating disorder. Often, they were also responsible for a fight or injuries caused to the inmates. Therefore, the asylum staff was not allowed to carry any sharp objects into the premises. At the Cuttack Lunatic Asylum, there was an accident in 1868. It was a fatal assault on a warder by an inmate. Since then no gardening tools were placed in the hands of patients.[33] According to the Superintendent of the Dullunda Asylum, keepers, both male and female, by their officious and meddlesome interference, often provoked unruliness among the inmates, which it was otherwise their duty to quell. Therefore, according to the officiating Superintending Surgeon, it was the establishment that required much more care and management than the patients.[34] Attendants' negligence of duties often resulted in fatal consequences, for instance, in 1872 at the Cuttack Lunatic Asylum, one 'imbecile' patient with the help of another committed suicide by hanging himself in his cell at night.[35] At the Dullunda Asylum, one patient drowned and another died from the rupture of the spleen, which, according to the duperintendent, happened because of ill treatment by an asylum staff

[31] General Proceedings, Medical Department, Number 4, January 1862, 'Report of the Moydapore Lunatic Asylum for the Year 1861,' WBSA.

[32] H. C. Cutcliffe, 'Report on the Dacca Lunatic Asylum for the Year 1869,' sent to Dr Buckle, Officiating Deputy Inspector General of Hospitals, Dacca Circle, dated 21 January 1871, *Annual Report on the Insane Asylums in Bengal for the Year 1869.*

[33] Home, Public, Medical, 1871, Annual Report to the Secretary to the Government of Bengal from Inspector General of Hospitals to J. Campbell Brown, Inspector General of Hospitals, Indian Medical Department, Fort William, dated 13 July 1871, NAI.

[34] R. Bird, 'Report on the Dullunda Lunatic Asylum for the Year 1872,' dated 24 April 1873, *Report on the Insane Asylums of Bengal for the Year 1872.*

[35] H. Cayley, 'Report on the Cuttack Lunatic Asylum for the Year 1872,' *Annual Report on the Insane Asylums of Bengal for the Year 1872.*

member who was assisted by two inmates. The person was convicted by the Sessions Court, and sentenced for rigorous imprisonment for four years. One case of suicide was recorded at Dacca and another at Patna. In each of the instances, the staff on duty was punished for carelessness. In another instance, when two criminal inmates escaped, one from Dacca and the other from Berhampore, one staff member was dismissed and several others were fined for negligence of duty.[36]

In certain asylums, no complaints against the 'native' establishment were registered. For instance, in the Patna Lunatic Asylum in 1862, according to John Balfour, Deputy Inspector General of Hospitals, the establishment, including the daroga, 'native' doctor, jemadars, and keepers, performed their duties in a very satisfactory way, and were careful and attentive at all times.[37]

The attendants were particularly cautious before medical officials visited the asylum for inspection. They were so particular about it that at Dullunda Asylum in 1865, during the superintendent's visiting hours, there was no trace of filth even in the rooms for inmates of filthy habits. The superintendent was very suspicious about it. He believed that the staff had made an added effort to specially clean the wards for their visits, which he doubted they would do under normal circumstances. According to Superintendent A. Payne, the

cleanliness is enforced to the utmost limits of reason and sometimes a little beyond them. Even a close smell in a room when the outer air is still, is treated as a fault and duly expiated by the sweepers on pay day.[38]

In contrast to the 'native' asylums, the superintendents of the European Lunatic Asylum were usually satisfied with the performance of the asylum staff. The Superintendent of the Bhawanipore Asylum mentioned in 1870 that the head Overseer and the matron were thoroughly suited in every respect to their duties and the daily routine of

[36] Municipal Department, Medical Branch, July 1896, Resolution Number 2960, 'Report on the Lunatic Asylums of Bengal for the Year 1895,' by H. H. Risley, Secretary to the Government of Bengal, APAC, BL.

[37] John Balfour, 'Report on the Patna Lunatic Asylum for the Year 1862,' *Annual Reports and Returns of the Insane Asylums in Bengal for the Years 1862–66.*

[38] A. Payne, 'Annual Report of the Dullunda Lunatic Asylum,' sent to H. M. Macpherson, Secretary, Principal Inspector General, Medical Department, dated 8 February 1866, *Annual Reports and Returns of the Insane Asylums in Bengal for the Years 1862–66.*

discipline and order was carried on almost without his intervention. Except during instances of acute cases that required medical treatment, his daily visit included the management of correspondence and other external business of the institution.[39] The management of the Bhawanipore Lunatic Asylum was always carefully and ably conducted. The comfort of the inmates was also thoroughly attended to, and the state of the asylum and appearance of the inmates indicated, according to Robert Bird, that they received all the necessary attention they needed. The patients at the asylum spent their time leisurely. This was partly attributed by the European physicians to the climatic condition which disposed European inmates to idleness, and partly to the disease from which the patients suffered. It was of less intensity than it was in Europe. Books and newspapers, and various indoor games, were at the disposal of the inmates. The compound and the interior of the asylum was cleaned and whitewashed: a dirty spot was barely visible anywhere. The Overseer and the matron, according to the superintendent, successfully managed to deal with the 'crude and insufficient' conditions of the toilet.[40]

By 1889, the lack of adequate staff in the 'native' asylums, due to the meagre salary, caused 'inconvenience and discomfort to the lunatics'.[41] Under such circumstances, the Inspector General was averse to a further reduction in the number of warders at any of the asylums. The pay of keepers at Patna and Berhampore Asylums was fixed at a uniform rate of Rs 6 a month. The amount was insufficient to attract 'good men'. Therefore, he recommended that the pay scale be revised for better recruitments.[42] But the problem was that the scarcity of staff in

[39] 'Report on the Insane Hospital at Bhawanipore,' sent to the Deputy Inspector General of Hospitals, Presidency Circle from the Superintendent of Asylums, Presidency, Fort William, Bhawanipore, dated February 1870, *Annual Report on the Insane Asylums in Bengal for the Year 1869*.

[40] R. Bird, 'Report on the Bhawanipore Lunatic Asylum for the Year 1872,' Fort William, Bhawanipore, dated 17 April 1873, *Annual Report on the Insane Asylums of Bengal for the Year 1872*.

[41] Home, Medical, Number 135, July 1890, 'Report on the Lunatic Asylums of Bengal for the Year 1889,' sent to the Chief Secretary of the Government of Bengal from A. Hilson, Inspector General of Civil Hospitals, Bengal, Calcutta, dated 8 April 1890, NAI.

[42] Home, Medical, Number 135, July 1890, 'Report on the Lunatic Asylums of Bengal for the Year 1889,' NAI.

the asylums was often substituted by the added labour of the inmates, thereby making them the victim of the situation.

Patients were sent outside the asylum during their occasional outings under the charge of the attendants. By 1898, selected patients were sent under proper escort to the zoological gardens in Calcutta. At Dacca, inmates were allowed to go to the bazaar and fields under the supervision of the keepers. Similarly, at Cuttack and Berhampore, patients were allowed to go outside the asylum in the custody of the attendants. At Patna, however, the patients were not allowed to go outside the asylum because the asylum was centrally located and the neighbourhood, according to T. H. Hendeley was 'overcrowded and unsanitary'.[43] In this context John Conolly had rightly pointed out:

> Means of amusements out of doors are useful to the attendants as well as to the patients; they contribute to relieve the irksomeness of their duties, and act as inducements to their taking the patients out as often as they can.[44]

DUTIES OF THE 'NATIVE' DOCTOR AND THE 'NATIVE' AND EUROPEAN OVERSEERS

Although the 'native' doctor and the 'native' and European Overseers were part of the establishment, their duties were of different kinds. Overseers were appointed for supervising the overall functioning of the establishment. The 'native' doctor was in charge of treatment of inmates apart from managing the establishment. The medical officers considered a European official more appropriate for the post of the Overseer as they did not find the 'native' trustworthy. Therefore, in 1860, a proposal was submitted for the appointment of a European Overseer in each of the lunatic asylums of the Lower Provinces.[45] In 1866, the Overseer and

[43] T. H. Hendeley, 'Report on the Lunatic Asylums of Bengal,' sent to the Secretary of the Government of Bengal, dated 14 March 1899, *Annual Report on the Lunatic Asylums of Bengal for the Year 1898*, by Colonel T. H. Hendeley, Inspector General of Civil Hospitals, Bengal (Calcutta: Bengal Secretariat Press, 1899), NAI.

[44] John Conolly, *The Construction and Government of Lunatic Asylums* (London: John Churchill, 1847), 54.

[45] Home, Public Proceedings, Medical, Bengal, Number 42, Enclosure in letter from T. Cantor to Secretary to the Director General of the Medical Department, 24 October 1859.

the 'native' doctor were placed in charge of the supervision of the daily tasks of the establishment. If an inmate refused to finish his meal, it was reported to the medical officers by the attendants.[46]

The medical officials were doubtful about the qualifications of the 'native' doctor. A. Fleming criticized the 'native' doctor of the Moorshedabad Asylum as an 'un passed' man who lacked the qualifications of a good 'native' doctor. Although he criticized him, he did not remove the doctor from his post. This was because the 'native' doctor had been attached to the asylum for a long time and had gained experience in the management of the insane. The anxiety over losing the 'native' doctor showed that they were not only in demand, but the European medical officers also depended on them. Therefore, the Civil Surgeon proposed to increase his pay from Rs 16 to Rs 20 per month in consideration of his long service since 1846, and the near 'prison life he led at the asylum without any leaves'.[47] In another instance, in 1869, the Superintendent decided to remove the 'native' doctor from his post because of negligence and also because of the unfavourable report that he had received against the doctor. He was replaced by Sheikh Bahadur, another 'native' man, who according to the superintendent, bore a good character in the military service, and who deserved the post. But he also expressed his misgivings about Sheikh Bahadur, who, according to him, did not have the necessary training that was required to administer the inmates in an asylum. He was also disappointed with the 'native' doctor because of the way he performed the duties of the asylum. Irrespective of the complaints that he had against Sheikh Bahadur, he did not remove him from the post because Sheikh Bahadur had earned the certificate of a well-recognized regimental 'native' doctor.[48]

Often, there were disagreements between two European officials over the appointment and performance of the asylum staff. For instance, the Deputy Inspector General of the Presidency Circle, G. Saunders,

[46] A. Payne, 'Annual Report of the Dullunda Lunatic Asylum' sent to H. M. Macpherson, 8 February 1866.

[47] A. Fleming, 'Report on the Moorshedabad Lunatic Asylum for the Year 1862'.

[48] A. Payne, 'Report on the Dullunda Lunatic Asylum for the Year 1869,' sent to the Deputy Inspector General of Hospitals, Presidency Circle, NAI.

disagreed with the superintendent of the asylum on the views of the conduct of the 'native' doctor Sheikh Bahadur. According to him, the 'native' doctor was an excellent human being and was selected by him because of his exceptionally good conduct and character. He was appointed to the asylum in place of a man who was 'notoriously inefficient and untrustworthy'.[49] Saunders believed that Sheikh Bahadur would prove himself worthy of the post in due course of time.[50]

The Surgeon Major of the Moorshedabad Asylum was full of admiration for the good conduct of Sergeant Frawley, the European Overseer, who was a steady, sober, and efficient officer. Frawley, according to him, also adapted well to the 'natives' with his even temper and knowledge of 'native' character. In contrast, the 'native servants', according to the Surgeon, were a constant source of trouble and annoyance, and were only the 'scum' of Berhampore.[51]

In one instance, there was a complaint against the European Overseer for sexual assault on a female inmate. In 1869, upon receiving charge of the Patna Lunatic Asylum the Superintending Surgeon received an unfavourable report about Overseer Manson from his forerunner. The Overseer's subsequent conduct also proved him to be completely unfit and unqualified. He fell ill within two months of joining his duty. Shortly after returning to duty, he was charged with 'committing a criminal assault upon a lunatic woman',[52] which could not be proved due to lack of evidence. But according to the superintendent, strong reasons existed for suspecting his conduct. Therefore, an order was issued for his removal. Although he was held back for some time

[49] Memorandum by the Deputy Inspector General of Hospitals, G. Saunders, Presidency Circle, in forwarding the Report to the Inspector General of Hospitals, Number 3385, dated 19 February 1870, appended to 'Report on the Dullunda Lunatic Asylum for the Year 1869,' sent to the Deputy Inspector General of Hospitals, Presidency Circle from A. Payne, NAI.

[50] Memorandum by the Deputy Inspector General of Hospitals, G. Saunders, Presidency Circle, in forwarding the Report to the Inspector General of Hospitals, Number 3385, dated 19 February 1870.

[51] A. Fleming, 'Report on the Moorshedabad Lunatic Asylum,' dated 8 February 1866, NAI.

[52] J. Bedford, 'Report of the Patna Lunatic Asylum,' sent to the Deputy Inspector General of Hospitals, Dinapore Circle, Patna, dated 1 January 1870, *Annual Report on the Insane Asylums in Bengal for the Year 1869.*

till his successor arrived, his immediate dismissal became mandatory owing to his disgraceful and insubordinate manner. The superintendent regretted the fact that the entire establishment got disorganized because of his conduct. This incident finally led to his replacement by a 'native' Overseer.[53] Although the medical officers considered 'natives' untrustworthy of any post, his replacement with a 'native' Overseer is worthy of note. The European Overseer, who was thought to be a 'good' man, therefore, damaged the gentlemanly, noble image of the civilizer. Once such an incident was registered, the European officials had no other option but to condemn the situation and replace him with a 'native' man. It was easier for the ruling class to take necessary legal steps against a 'native' man than against a European who upheld an image of racial superiority.

In another instance, the European Overseer was suspended because he had quarrelled with the whole of the establishment, and particularly with the 'native' doctor. According to the superintendent, the 'native' doctor was a useful and attentive man, but eventually he also became 'insubordinate and insolent'. Finally, he too was suspended and was 'sent to a distant and inferior post as a punishment'. The 'native' doctor appointed in his place proved satisfactory, as did the 'native' Overseer or daroga who was placed temporarily in charge of the asylum until the arrival of a European Overseer who was transferred from Cuttack. The superintendent believed that things would improve under the superintendence of the latter, and also proposed to appoint the European Overseer's wife in charge of the female ward.[54]

In 1869, under the supervision of the European Overseer of the Cuttack Lunatic Asylum, Mr Nowlan, nearly all the clothing used in the asylum was manufactured by the inmates. Although his salary caused a considerable increase in the median expense for each patient, the superintendent was of opinion, quite without grounds, that European supervision was most urgently required in an asylum. The superintendent believed that the Government would also realize the necessity of

[53] J. Bedford, 'Report of the Patna Lunatic Asylum,' *Annual Report on the Insane Asylums in Bengal for the Year 1869.*

[54] Report of Deputy Inspector General H. M. Macpherson Appended to 'Report of the Patna Lunatic Asylum' from Surgeon J. Bedford, *Annual Report on the Insane Asylums in Bengal for the Year 1869.*

sanctioning another European Overseer to the Cuttack Asylum, because during an emergency or a violent and sudden outburst amongst inmates, he did not find 'native' supervision reliable.[55]

Although Freeman, Overseer of the Dullunda Asylum, suffered from a severe and dangerous illness, which was due to his daily exposure to the hot season since his employment, according to the superintendent, there was no abatement of his ever-ready and intelligent activity. He was a man of 'exemplary' character and 'diligence', and singularly full of 'tact and temper'[56] in controlling the 'native' establishment and the patients. He was also described as active and vigilant in directing the work in progress. He worked throughout the year without a fault or failure.[57] At the Dacca Lunatic Asylum, the Overseer, Mr Blackwell, was devoted to the poor patients in the asylum for which he received favourable recognition and reward from the Superintendent as well. The 'native' doctor Sheikh Kurreem Bux was also reported to be kind to the inmates, and attentive to his duties.[58]

By the 1870s, 'native' Overseers were also appointed in place of European Overseers. European medical officers considered the 'natives' as unable to examine the proper functioning of the asylum. While the European medical officers did not approve of the 'native' asylum staff, they could not fully disapprove of them either. For instance, at Cuttack, Dr Cayley reported that the performance of both the 'native' daroga and warder was agreeable. The 'native' Overseer, Sheikh Imamuddin, and eight warders appointed under him, performed their duties satisfactorily. They treated inmates with kindness, and also managed them firmly and judiciously.[59]

[55] J. MacDonald, 'Report on the Cuttack Lunatic Asylum for the Year 1869,' sent to the Secretary Inspector General of Hospitals, Indian Medical Department, Calcutta, dated 12 January 1870, *Annual Report on the Insane Asylums in Bengal for the Year 1869*.

[56] A. Payne, 'Annual Report of the Dullunda Lunatic Asylum for the Year 1862,' sent to H. M. Macpherson, *Annual Reports and Returns of the Insane Asylums in Bengal for the Years 1862–66*.

[57] A. Payne, 'Annual Report of the Dullunda Lunatic Asylum for the Year 1862,' sent to H. M. Macpherson, *Annual Reports and Returns of the Insane Asylums in Bengal for the Years 1862–66*.

[58] H. C. Cutcliffe, 'Report on the Dacca Lunatic Asylum for the Year 1869,' sent to Dr Buckle, Officiating Deputy Inspector General of Hospitals, Dacca Circle, NAI.

[59] H. Cayley, 'Report on the Cuttack Lunatic Asylum for the Year 1872,' *Annual Report on the Insane Asylums of Bengal for the Year 1872*.

At the same time at the Moydapore Asylum, the daroga and other workers of the establishment were commended because they were 'careful and deserving'. According to the superintendent, the daroga was unremitting in his care and attention, and most praiseworthy in carrying out every order given to him. The Committee was pleased with his duties and recommended a gradual increase in his salary. When initiatives were taken at Moydapore Asylum to educate 'lunatics', the daroga and the 'native' doctor were placed in charge of it. They efficiently established and supervised education among the inmates. The 'native' doctor also obtained special attention of the superintendent because he was considered as attentive, not only to the sick, but also in making himself generally useful among the inmates of the Moydapore Asylum. The superintendent was sympathetic and described his work as more anxious, confining, and unpleasant than that of 'native' doctors in charge of dispensaries who received Rs 40, which was double his pay.[60]

On the issue of the appointment of a 'native' over a European Overseer, the Superintendent Surgeon of the Cuttack Lunatic Asylum in 1871 stated that the 'native' Overseer appointed in the asylum was a good man but at the same time he also regretted the removal of the European Overseer from the asylum. According to him, 'natives' were all very well when looked after, but in an emergency they were unable to think and supervise. He further stated that under such circumstances they treated the troublesome inmates with severity. Hence, he strongly recommended the reappointment of a European Overseer in the Cuttack Asylum.[61]

At Dacca, the conduct of both the European Overseer and the 'native' doctor were commended by the superintendent. The Deputy Inspector General of Hospitals was satisfied with Mr Camilliri, the kind, attentive, and judicious Overseer of the asylum, because he took an interest in the manufactures of the asylum, and encouraged inmates to be industrious. In 1872, there were no reports of deaths caused by accident, although there were reports about a few injuries, which were inflicted by the patients on one another. The superintendent credited the European Overseer for his good conduct in dealing with such situations, but also admitted that it

[60] J. M. Coates, 'Report on the Moydapore Lunatic Asylum for the Year 1872,' *Annual Report on the Insane Asylums of Bengal for the Year 1872.*

[61] A. Fleming, 'Report on the Cuttack Lunatic Asylum for the Year 1871,' *Annual Report on the Insane Asylums in Bengal for the Year 1871.*

showed that the care exercised by the asylum staff towards the patients had become more constant than before. The government even sanctioned him a reward, which was paid from the industrial fund.[62]

The 'native' doctor Prosono Commar Sen performed much more laborious duties than other 'native' doctors of his standing, and received only two-thirds of their pay. Yet he continued to work and was in attendance day and night at the asylum. The superintendent was apprehensive about his stay at the asylum, because his companions in charge of district dispensaries received Rs 40. Therefore, he wanted the 'native' doctor's pay to also be increased from Rs 25 to Rs 40 a month.[63] The 'native' doctor's task was to keep the inmates under constant observation so that any form of illness could be attended to in its earliest stage.[64]

The total size of the asylum staff appointed at the Dullunda Asylum was inadequate to control the large number of inmates. The resident European Overseer managed 340 patients in 1871 with the assistance of the 'native' servants under him. Therefore, he failed to meet the expected demands. The solution was to reduce the number of inmates or to reconstitute the establishment altogether. According to A. Payne, the Superintending Surgeon, large populous asylums were universally condemned in England as the site of many evils. He further stated that on no account should more than 250 patients be assembled together under any system of management, and even that was an excessive number with establishments such as those of Bengal. Although the Surgeon considered the European Overseer as active and intelligent, he expressed his doubts about his capabilities when he stated that any mishap, due to his negligence, would ruin the reputation of the institution 'before public'.[65] European medical officials

[62] James Wise, 'Report on Dacca Lunatic Asylum,' *Annual Report on the Insane Asylums of Bengal for the Year 1872.*

[63] James Wise, 'Report on Dacca Lunatic Asylum,' *Annual Report on the Insane Asylums of Bengal for the Year 1872.*

[64] Memorandum number 1514, from H. B. Buckle, Deputy Inspector General of Hospital, Dacca Circle, to the Secretary to the Inspector General of Hospitals, Indian Medical Department, Shillong, dated 13 February 1873, *Annual Report on the Insane Asylums of Bengal for the Year 1872.*

[65] Home, Public, Medical Department, Number 19, 17 August 1871, Letter sent to the Officiating Secretary to the Government of Bengal, Judicial Department from A. Payne, Superintendent of Asylums at the Presidency, letter number 281, Fort William, Dullunda, dated 4 August 1871, APAC, BL.

not only doubted the capability of a 'native' Overseer, a European Overseer was also not exempted from such criticisms. It was necessary for them to be particular about the dignified image of the Europeans appointed for the post.

At the Dullunda Asylum, both the European Overseer and the matron received the special attention of the Superintendent. The Overseer, Mr Bancroft, worked for the welfare of the inmates. His post was considered as a difficult one because the institution by the 1870s was at the same time a hospital and a jail, where the patients required far more attention, care, and management.[66]

DUTIES OF WOMEN STAFF MEMBERS

This could be divided into two categories: first, the female staff members appointed from outside the asylum for the post of attendant, keeper, and matron; second, female patients who were recruited as asylum staff from within. European women were specifically appointed for the post of the matron. They were commended for their tactful approach towards the inmates. Although appointment to the post did not have any necessary criteria, it was expected by the European officers that other than providing them with information on female patients they would also help to impart 'feminine lessons' to them. 'Native' women were probably not thought of ideal for the post, not only because of the medical officers' general suspicion towards them but also because of the fact that such an appointment had a missionary approach to healing as well, where a brown woman was taken care of and disciplined by a white woman.

At Dullunda Asylum in 1866, a European matron was appointed at the pay of Rs 50 per month, so that the superintendent could get a detailed report on female inmates, which had been otherwise not possible earlier in the absence of any female matron.[67] The late matron of the European Lunatic Asylum, Mrs De Vere, was known to have engaged female patients in sewing and knitting during the day time.

[66] R. Bird, 'Report on the Dullunda Lunatic Asylum for the Year 1872,' *Report on the Insane Asylums of Bengal for the Year 1872.*

[67] R. Bird, 'Report on the Dullunda Lunatic Asylum for the Year 1872,' *Report on the Insane Asylums of Bengal for the Year 1872.*

According to the superintendent, the matron Mrs De Vere, with her tact and kindliness of heart, won the trust of the patients and was successful in managing the patients. Mrs Hamilton, who succeeded as matron after her mother Mrs De Vere's death, was also known to be attentive to the welfare of the patients.[68] Mrs Monteiro, the matron of Dullunda Asylum was also known to have done her work quietly, steadily, and effectively, and under her care women were well looked after and discreetly managed.[69]

Usually 'native' female attendants were appointed for female inmates. But amongst the female patients of the Dullunda Asylum appointed as asylum staff,[70] there were both 'native' and Eurasian women. At times, Eurasian or Anglo-Indian women were sent back from the European Lunatic Asylum to the 'native' asylums instead of sending them back to England. European Lunatic Asylum, as per their asylum rule, only took charge of sending European lunatics back to England. Female patients did not have any place to return to once they were cured; in these cases they were usually absorbed in various asylum jobs. Table 4.1 shows a list of cured 'lunatic' women of the Dullunda Asylum and the relevant job in which they were employed into.[71]

The employment of female staff for the patients continued to be the same until the end of the nineteenth century when dhais were encouraged for the post instead of mehtarnees.[72] There were instances of women giving birth in the European Lunatic Asylum and their children being sent to the Orphan School of Calcutta. But there were no such references in case of 'native' women. Therefore, the appointment of such posts illustrated a significant change in the management

[68] R. Bird, 'Report on the Dullunda Lunatic Asylum for the Year 1872,' *Report on the Insane Asylums of Bengal for the Year 1872*.

[69] R. Bird, 'Report on the Dullunda Lunatic Asylum for the Year 1872,' *Report on the Insane Asylums of Bengal for the Year 1872*.

[70] Home, Public, Medical Department, Number 19, Letter from A. Payne to Officiating Secretary to the Government of Bengal, 4 August 1871.

[71] Home, Public, Medical Department, Number 19, Letter from A. Payne to Officiating Secretary to the Government of Bengal, 4 August 1871.

[72] Municipal Department, Medical Branch, Number 15, February 1900, Copy of Remarks made by Surgeon T. H. Hendeley, Inspector General of Civil Hospitals on his visit to the Dacca Lunatic Asylum, dated 26 July 1898, APAC, BL.

Table 4.1 List of 'Recovered' Women Patients Who Were Employed in Various Duties in the Dullunda Asylum

Name	Employment
Badsha Bebee	In cleaning rooms
Boba (unknown)	In cleaning rooms
Rajee Kamenee	In cleaning rooms
Mary Ann Williams	In cleaning rooms
Munmohenee	As goorgeen
Marian	As goorgeen
Soondry	As mehtarnee

Source: Home, Public, Medical Department, Number 19, Letter from A. Payne to Officiating Secretary to the Government of Bengal, 4 August 1871.

of female inmates. It showed that mehtarnees initially performed the duty of delivering babies inside the asylum. Although official records did not mention any woman delivering in the asylum, but the appointment of dhais, who played a significant role in delivering babies, clearly indicated that such incidents were prevalent in the 'native' asylums. Given that there was no scope of knowing whether these women came already pregnant into the asylum or got pregnant while admitted there made the situation difficult. In case of the latter occurrence, it became mandatory on the part of the European officials to take necessary action. This was because by the late nineteenth century, with the growing importance of imperialism and with notions of motherhood and the popularity of the Dufferin Fund in India, motherhood was valorized, and child birth seen as crucial in the life of a woman.

THE MANAGEMENT AND PAY OF THE ESTABLISHMENT

The duty of the asylum staff was fixed but there was no appropriate provision for their pay. Therefore, throughout the nineteenth century there were discussions about the management and pay of asylum staff. This situation worsened so much over time that by the late nineteenth century, the asylum staff expressed its resentment and often left their asylum jobs in search of a 'better paid' job elsewhere.

In 1817, according to the rules established for the management and control of the 'native' insane hospitals[73] the establishment consisted of a 'native' doctor who was appointed at a salary of Rs 16. He resided within the compound and worked under the order of the Surgeon. At the head of establishment was a daroga or head 'native' keeper who received a monthly salary of Rs 10. He worked under the control and direction of the medical officers. The head 'native' keeper was in charge of the general management of the patients and held authority over other members of the establishment. In the male ward of the asylums one *naib* jemadar or deputy keeper was appointed on a salary of Rs 8 for every thirty patients. And for every eight patients, a peon, coolie, or negaban was appointed at the cost of Rs 4. One mehtar was appointed on a wage of Rs 3 or Rs 4 for every twenty patients and one barber was appointed for every fifty patients at the cost of Rs 3. The salary of the barber was the lowest because his service was occasional. Female patients had one head woman keeper at Rs 6 per month, one female coolie at Rs 4 for every eight inmates, and one mehetarnee or sweeper for every twenty patients. One cook was appointed for every forty inmates, both male and female, at the cost of Rs 5. One guala or Hindu water carrier was appointed to carry water to the cook room for Hindu patients at the cost of Rs 4.[74] The appointment of a Hindu water carrier illustrated the fact that there was a distinct division among patients on the basis of caste and community, unlike in the European Lunatic Asylum where the division was based on class. One dhobi was appointed at the cost of Rs 5 for every fifty patients. Finally, one harkara was appointed at the cost of Rs 4 for carrying messages and in cases where the asylum grounds were extensive, one or two malis were appointed at the cost of Rs 4 each.[75]

In 1820, the Medical Board empowered the Magistrate with the right to increase or diminish the size of the staff. The Magistrate, after consulting the Surgeon of the asylum, increased or diminished the scale of payment or varied its distribution. In order to determine the number of asylum staff and their pay, the establishment was occasionally inspected by him. Under such circumstances, the Civil Surgeon of Moorshedabad

[73] *Rules for the Management and Control of the Native Insane Hospitals* (Calcutta: Baptist Mission Press, 1825), 1–12, NL.

[74] *Rules for the Management and Control of the Native Insane Hospitals*, 1–12.

[75] *Rules for the Management and Control of the Native Insane Hospitals*, 1–12.

Asylum, in 1820, appealed to the Magistrate requesting him to grant the permission to maintain a permanent and fixed establishment. Instead of increasing or diminishing the number he requested the Magistrate to allow him to maintain the same establishment as it existed at Moorshedabad Asylum. This was not only because the establishment acquired the trust of the superintendent but also because he considered the existing establishment as experienced and trained in managing patients.[76]

While the number of staff members and their pay were decided by the Magistrate, the internal management of the establishment was placed under the control and order of the medical officers. For instance, it was the Surgeon's duty to inspect the attendants so that they abstained from all acts of oppression and unnecessary severity towards the lunatics. Therefore, without his instruction attendants were not allowed to use irons, straitjackets, waistcoats, or any other form of restraints. Under all circumstances, they were expected by the medical officials to be mild, patient, and humane. According to Tuke, no attendant was permitted to strike a patient, or address him in violent language or in a loud tone. He further stated that the proportion of attendants to patients 'must be materially increased in those asylums in which the strait waistcoat' and other forms of mechanical restraints were completely abolished.[77] This proportion was never achieved in the asylums of Bengal, irrespective of the fact whether restraint was abolished or not.

The role of the asylum staff was an indispensable part of the asylum management. While other members of the establishment looked after the maintenance of the asylum, the attendants' duty was to look after the care, treatment, security, and welfare of the patients. Throughout the nineteenth century, any proposal for a new asylum was appended with a list of the members of the establishment and their monthly wages. For instance, during the establishment of the 'native' Insane Hospital at Calcutta, the monthly allowance proposed[78] by the Magistrate for the

[76] Medical Board Proceedings, Number 18, 24 October 1820, Enclosure attached to the letter sent to James Jameson, Secretary Medical Board from W. B. Bayley, Chief Secretary to Government, NAI.

[77] Tuke, *Moral Management of the Insane*, 100–1.

[78] Bengal, Criminal and Judicial Proceedings, 1 November 1819, Number 19, Enclosure attached to a letter sent to George Dowdeswell, Secretary to Government by John Eliot, Tipperah Magistrate, APAC, BL.

'native establishment' included Rs 16 for the 'native' doctor, Rs 10 for jemadar, Rs 32 in total for eight peons—which came to an average of Rs 4 per peon—Rs 10 for two cooks, Rs 8 for two matrons, Rs 8 for two bheesties; the total amounted to Rs 84.[79]

The situation was different in the European Lunatic Asylum at Bhawanipore. The establishment proposed by the Medical Board for the European Asylum in 1817, consisted of two European male attendants or keepers, one for the upper ranks and another for the lower rank of inmates, whereas only one female attendant was appointed for the female patients of all ranks. These three attendants worked under the immediate control and supervision of the Surgeon of the hospital and his assistant. The attendants were paid a monthly salary of Rs 80 per head and quarters were provided to accommodate them within the compound. Along with this, two 'native' head attendants, one for male and another for female patients were also appointed for the upper-class inmates at the cost of Rs 12 per month. The Department of Commissariat was responsible for the payment of the asylum staff in the European Lunatic Asylum as most of the inmates admitted there were soldiers. The establishment was regularly visited on the first day of each month by the visiting member of the Medical Board whose duty was to ascertain the regular maintenance of the entire establishment.[80]

In April 1835, the Medical Board in a letter to the Governor recommended a certain number of attendants necessary for the asylums, which the Board considered sufficient for the custody and safe maintenance of patients in Russapaglah, Dacca, Moorshedabad, and Patna asylums. As per these recommendations, the attendants for every twenty four male lunatics who were admitted from the Regiments included: one Surgeon, one 'native' doctor, one daroga, and one naib or a deputy, along with one peon for every five patients. For non-Regimental cases, one naib was appointed for every twenty patients, one peon for every six patients, and in case of both Regimental and non-Regimental

[79] Medical Board Proceedings, 31 January 1821, Number 21 B, Enclosure attached to a letter sent to W. Ogilvy, President and Member of the Medical Board by C. Lushington, Secretary to Government in General Department, dated 28 June 1820, NAI.

[80] Medical Board Proceedings, Enclosure attached to Letter from C. Lushington to W. Ogilvy, 28 June 1820.

patients, one mehtar was appointed for every fifteen patients, and there was one barber for every fifty inmates. The asylum staff appointed for female patients included one female keeper, one female coolie for every six patients, and one mehtarnee for every fifteen patients. The common establishment for both male and female inmates included: one cook for every forty patients, one bheesty for every forty patients, one guala, one dhobi for every fifty patients, one harkara, and one mali for the garden attached to the hospital who also assisted inmates in gardening.[81] The Governor stated in reply that unless the proportion of attendants to the patients was found insufficient in practice, the government was not bound to increase either the number of servants in the establishment or their expenses. Instead, he proposed to maintain the number of attendants that already existed, for example, one mehtar appointed for every twenty-six patients rather than to every fifteen patients.[82] The Board in course of its further correspondence with the government stated that they were 'misapprehended by government'. The former actually suggested for a considerable reduction instead of an increase in expense.[83]

Although the demand was for reduction of attendants, the medical officer in charge of the Russapaglah Hospital appealed for the reverse. The Surgeon of the Insane Hospital, F. P Strong, stated that reductions could be fatal for the care of the inmates. In December 1835, Strong sent a letter to the government through the Magistrate of the 24 Parganas proposing changes to the plan suggested by the Medical Board of placing all insane institutions upon a uniform footing with respect to establishment, clothing, and diet.[84] Although the Government tried

---

[81] Medical Board Proceedings, Number 7, 13 April 1835, Letter sent to C. J. Metcalf, Governor of Bengal in Council from the Members of the Medical Board, dated 10 April 1835, NAI.

[82] Medical Board Proceedings, Number 18, 15 June 1835, Letter sent to the Medical Board from Mr. Mangles, Secretary to the Government of Bengal in the Judicial Department, dated 6 June 1835, NAI.

[83] Medical Board Proceedings, Number 9, 18 June 1835, Letter number 174, letter sent to the Governor of Bengal in Council by Langstaff and Swiney, Members of the Medical Board, Medical Board Office, dated 17 June 1835, NAI.

[84] Medical Board Proceedings, Number 11, 21 December 1835, Enclosure attached to a letter sent to the Medical Board from Mr Mangles, Secretary to Government, dated 15 December 1835, NAI.

to maintain uniformity in the number and pay of attendants in all the 'native' asylums of Bengal, as per the rule set up in 1819, it reduced to half the number by 1829. Lack of funds to support the establishment further complicated the situation.

The 'native' establishment was indispensable for the maintenance of inmates while at the same time the government was not willing to increase their pay. For instance, in 1831, one rupee was deducted from the pay of the head female keeper who worked in the Insane Hospital at Russapaglah since 1804. Until 1819, she had received a sum of Rs 6 every month.[85]

According to the Surgeon of the hospital, if the 'lunatics' were to be discharged from the asylums sooner and taken care of at their homes, the monthly expenses of the government for the maintenance of attendants could be reduced.[86] This proposal was problematic. First, this would put the asylum officials at a haste to treat patients; second, while this kind of a proposition was applicable in case of lunatics in the European Lunatic Asylum where families, friends, or relatives paid for the maintenance of the patients in the asylum, it was not possible for patients at the 'native' lunatic asylums. Almost all of the 'lunatics' in the 'native' asylums of Bengal were maintained by the government and not by individuals. Therefore, once discharged, cured or not cured, they did not have a place to return to.

In 1829, as per the suggestion of the Medical Board, the Surgeon of Russapaglah reduced the number of mehtars to one quarter of the number, negabans or attendants were reduced to one half and the up-country naib jemadars were reduced to one third of their number. But as further reduction was proposed by 1831, the Surgeon insisted that number of naib jemadars should not be reduced. It was because the assistance of this physically strong class of attendants was essential in emergencies. He alluded to the opinion of the Commissioner Mr E. R. Barwell who also earnestly denounced any reduction. The Surgeon therefore, in a letter to the Sudder Nizamat Adalat (District Court) accentuated the necessity of an increase rather than a reduction in the number of attendants.

[85] Medical Board Proceedings, Number 11, Enclosure attached to Letter from Mr Mangles to the Medical Board, 15 December 1835.
[86] Medical Board Proceedings, Number 11, Enclosure attached to Letter from Mr Mangles to the Medical Board, 15 December 1835.

F. P. Strong did not consider the number of attendants, allowed in the printed rules for the management and control of the 'native' Insane Hospital formed in 1819, as sufficient for the duties required of them and for the safety of the patients.[87]

The reduction proposed by the Medical Board in 1835, included one peon for every ten patients who were previously allotted for every eight patients. Again, one mehtar was appointed for every twenty-six patients, which earlier this was for every twenty patients. However, the Board did not propose to reduce the number of 'native' doctors, jemadars, naib jemadars, cooks, bheesties, barbers, coolies, gualas, harkara, and malis, and hence, these continued to be the same.[88]

The point of difference in the rule of 1819 to that of 1829 as regards servants and attendants was that the total number of the workers of the establishment was reduced in 1829 from what existed earlier. This had put the management of patients in asylums at risk. Besides the already existing members of the establishment, the regulations of 1829 allowed one negaban peon to every five insane patients. Until the reduction in 1829, a larger number of them were also appointed at Russapaglah jail to control the insane prisoners.

According to the Surgeon, 'the reduction would have been considered sufficient and that a further attempt at reduction was not in contemplation rather than put any difficulty in the way of economy'.[89] Hence, until 1835, he too tried to implement such reductions in practice in the asylum even though he disagreed with them. He adopted the reduction of one negaban peon for every eight patients. But he changed his plan for further reduction when an accident took place in the asylum in which an insane villager died from a single blow when, on a stormy night, a rafter was thrust upon him by another mentally ill prisoner. The Surgeon pointed out that the removal of one night guard out of a total of two night guards had led to this disaster. He further stated that in 'sickly' seasons, by which he meant the hot and rainy months of the year, half

[87] Medical Board Proceedings, Number 11, Enclosure attached to Letter from Mr Mangles to the Medical Board, 15 December 1835.

[88] Medical Board Proceedings, Number 11, Enclosure attached to Letter from Mr Mangles to the Medical Board, 15 December 1835.

[89] Medical Board Proceedings, Number 11, Enclosure attached to Letter from Mr Mangles to the Medical Board, 15 December 1835.

the attendants were sick due to fever. Their duty was not only arduous at all times, it was particularly demanding during the 'sickly' seasons when many patients also fell sick.[90] Therefore, attendants were in high demand. The medical officials were against any reduction, because in the presence of the asylum staff it was always easier for them to treat a patient.

The number of staff members appointed at the jail was different from that of the asylum. Dr Strong, while referring to this difference, pointed out that in the jail, for every four convicts, one negaban peon was allowed as a day and night guard and one barkandaze similar to the naib jemadar of the asylum was appointed for every fifteen patients. In certain cases, the number of peons was increased by appointing one for every three prisoners. In the asylum one attendant was appointed for every five insane patients, violent or tranquil. The proportion of attendants to patients was one to five until it became one attendant for every eight 'lunatics' by 1835. The Surgeon was apprehensive of the proportion of attendants to patients. According to him, the small number of attendants was insufficient when cases of mental illness were extreme. Under such circumstances it was also unsafe to admit violent patients in the asylum. This was also approved of by the Civil Assistant Surgeon of the Moorshedabad Asylum, A. Kean. Although he tactfully expressed his satisfaction with the Board's proposal, he indicated the need for an increased proportion of attendants in case of an increase in the number of patients.[91]

Finally, by December 1835, the Governor of Bengal resolved to not make any alteration in the existing method of conducting the Insane Hospitals.[92] Therefore, the issue of the number of attendants was not resolved. While the Board demanded reductions, the Surgeons of the asylums demanded the opposite and the government was unwilling to consider either. The government's refusal to make necessary amendments not only revealed the problem of the lack of funds and their

[90] Medical Board Proceedings, Number 11, Enclosure attached to Letter from Mr Mangles to the Medical Board, 15 December 1835.

[91] Medical Board Proceedings, Number 11, Enclosure attached to Letter from Mr Mangles to the Medical Board, 15 December 1835.

[92] Medical Board Proceedings, Number 11, Enclosure attached to Letter from Mr Mangles to the Medical Board, 15 December 1835.

indifference towards the issue, it also showed that unlike medical officers of the asylums the government did not consider the issue over attendants seriously.

In 1858 under Section IX of Act XXXVI of 1858, new regulations were proposed for the maintenance of the establishment. According to the new regulations, the rate of bheesties was reduced to Rs 4 instead of its previous rate of Rs 5. The same rate was also proposed for the nega-bans.[93] This reduced rate complicated the situation as it became difficult to recruit either of them into the establishment. The medical officials were considerate about the position of the asylum staff, because they helped the officials to look after inmates and also provided information regarding them. Therefore, in several instances, the officials proposed to the government to increase both the number and salary of the staff. A. Payne, Superintendent of the Dullunda Asylum, proposed an increase in the pay because the task included a constant surveillance by the attendants of the patients.[94] Although he proposed an increase in pay, he was also strict about the proper functioning of the staff, as he also pointed out that in case of 'dereliction of duty' the establishment had to 'pay fine as punishment' (see Table 4.2).[95]

Other than the attendants, the asylum faced a similar crisis regarding peons and malis. In order to resolve the situation, an application was submitted to the government for a rate of not less than Rs 5 per month, at least for those staff members who were required to devote their entire time for the maintenance of the institution. The visitors of the Dullunda Asylum also proposed the recruitment of a *durwan* indispensable. Therefore, they recommended the appointment of a durwan on a rate similar to that at Bhawanipore Asylum, and further requested the superintendent of the asylum to apply, without delay, through the medical department for the

[93] Home, Public Proceedings, Medical, Bengal, Number 47, 19 July 1860, Letter sent to Assistant Surgeon N. Chevers, Secretary Principal Inspector General, Medical Department from Assistant Surgeon A. Payne, Superintendent Native Lunatic Asylum, Dullunda, letter number 97, dated 27 June 1860, APAC, BL.
[94] Home, Public Proceedings, Medical, Bengal, Number 47, Letter from A. Payne to N. Chevers, 27 June 1860.
[95] Home, Public Proceedings, Medical, Bengal, Number 47, Letter from A. Payne to N. Chevers, 27 June 1860.

Table 4.2 A Comparative Statement Showing the Existing Scale of Pay until 1860 and the New Proposed Scale of Establishment for the Asylum for 'Native' Insane Patients at Dullunda, near Fort William

Extract from Home Department, GoI	Office to which the Proposition Refers	Nature of Charges		Permanent Increase per Month	Grounds of Proposition
		Present Scale	Proposed Scale		
	Asylum for native insane, Dullunda	1 European Overseer Rs As P 10 0 0	Rs As P 10 0 0	–	The impossibility of procuring servants of the several classes in Calcutta at rates lower than those specified in the proposed scale, and the great inconvenience that is felt in an institution of this kind from the absconding of dissatisfied servants, this practice having become frequent of late from the high price of necessaries and the facilities that servants enjoy of getting more lucrative employment in other establishments than is now afforded to them in the asylum

(Cont'd)

Table 4.2 (*Cont'd*)

Extract from Home Department, GoI	Office to which the Proposition Refers	Nature of Charges		Permanent Increase per Month	Grounds of Proposition
		Present Scale	Proposed Scale		
		1 *naib* for every thirty male patients at Rs 10, say 8 in number 80 0 0	80 0 0	—	
		1 *negaben* for every 8 male patients at Rs 4, say 28 in number 112 0 0	Rs 5, say 28 140 0 0	28 0 0	
		1 cook for every 50 patients, say 6 in number at Rs 5 30 0 0	30 0 0		
		1 *bheesty* for every 40 patients, say 7 at Rs 4 28 0 0	Rs 5 35 0 0	7 0 0	
		1 Hindu water carrier 4 0 0	... 5 0 0	1 0 0	

1 *mehtar* for every 20 males, say 11 at Rs 4	Rs 5	55 0 0	11 0 0
44 0 0			
1 *harkara*	6	6 0 0	2 0 0
4 0 0			
2 gardeners at Rs 4	Rs 5		2 0 0
8 0 0	10 0 0		
1 barber for every 50 patients at Rs 3, say 5		15 0 0	–
15 0 0			
1 durwan, Rs 6	6 0 0		–
6 0 0			
1 female keeper	6 0 0		' –
6 0 0			
1 female *negaban* for every 8 patients, say 6, at Rs 4	... Rs 5		6 0 0
24 0 0	30 0 0		
1 *mehtarnee* for every 20 patients, say 2, at Rs 4	Rs 5		2 0 0
8 0 0	10 0 0		
Extra establishment	Extra establishment		

(Cont'd)

Table 4.2 (*Contd*)

Extract from Home Department, GoI	Office to which the Proposition Refers	Nature of Charges		Permanent Increase per Month	Grounds of Proposition
		Present Scale	Proposed Scale		
		1 lamp lighter			
		4 0 0	...	1 0 0	
			5 0 0		
		2 *bheesties* at Rs 5	10 0 0	–	
		10 0 0			
		1 head *mehtar*, at Rs 5	... Rs 6	1 0 0	
		5 0 0	6 0 0		
		4 *mehtars*, at Rs 4	... Rs 5	4 0 0	
		16 0 0	20 0 0		
		1 *mehtarnee*, at Rs 4	... Rs 5	1 0 0	
		4 0 0	5 0 0		
		Total 552 0 0	624 0 0	72 0 0	

Source: Home Department, Public Proceedings, Medical Branch, Bengal, Number 48, 19 July 1860, APAC, BL.

necessary orders. Although in 1860, new regulations empowered visitors in place of the Magistrates to increase or decrease the number of asylum staff, they did not have the authority to fix the wages of the new staff. Finally, the new regulations made no provision for a durwan, and therefore, one peon was employed in that place at Dullunda Asylum.[96] This showed that the administrative officials saw no difference between the role of a durwan or a peon. This uncertainty in formulating regulations instead created a class of people who were capable of doing their duties in whichever posts they were appointed to. It, therefore, created a situation in which the duties of the asylum staff were constantly overlapping and they often did not have a fixed duty to perform. A comparative statement showing the existing scale of pay until 1860 and the new proposed scale of establishment for the Dullunda Asylum is shown in Table 4.2.

In 1859, the pay scale of the 'native' establishment was proposed along with the plan of the Cuttack Asylum. The new scale was different from the one proposed in 1817 for all the 'native' asylums of Bengal. There was an increase in pay of the overall establishment. For instance, it recommended the hiring of one overseer at the cost of Rs 25, one 'native' doctor at the cost of Rs 20 instead of Rs 16, one jemadar at the cost of Rs 6, instead of Rs 5, four male attendants at Rs 4 each, one female attendant at Rs 4, one male cook at the cost of Rs 4, one female cook at Rs 4, one gardener at Rs 3, one washer man at Rs 4, and one sweeper at Rs 3; the total amounted to Rs 89. A small guard or a *naik* and eight men from the police battalion were also appointed to guard the outside of the asylum both during day and night.[97] Therefore, new regulations in the period following 1858 not only proposed a new scale of payment, but also introduced new posts within the establishment by incorporating specialized men from the police force for the management of mentally ill patients.

[96] Home, Public Proceedings, Medical, Bengal, Number 47, 19 July 1860, Extract from the Proceedings of the Visitors, Dullunda Lunatic Asylum at a Meeting held on 12 June 1860, Enclosed to a Letter sent to Assistant Surgeon N. Chevers, Secretary Principal Inspector General, Medical Department from Assistant Surgeon A. Payne, APAC, BL.

[97] Home, Public Proceedings, Medical, Bengal, Number 23, 5 April 1860, Letter sent to G. F. Cockburn, Commissioner of Cuttack to the Secretary to the Government of Bengal, Letter number 163, dated 6 September 1859. APAC, BL.

The appointment of staff differed from one asylum to another. At a time when the post of daroga was not sanctioned at Dullunda Asylum, the Surgeon of the Patna Asylum in 1860 proposed a monthly increase of pay of daroga, already appointed there, from Rs 10 to Rs 20. The reason for his proposal was that government servants serving at other institutions with similar qualifications received a higher scale of pay than in the asylum. Two jemadars previously appointed at the asylum received a pay of Rs 5 per month. Instead, he suggested an increase of Rs 5 for the senior jemadar, and Rs 3 for the junior jemadar.[98] This idea of a subdivision between similar posts was to put one in control over the other, thereby making the post more challenging.

The keepers, male and female, as well as the sweepers, received Rs 3 per month. The Surgeon disapproved of the amount, because he considered it inadequate to support the asylum staff. According to him, the price of food had doubled since the initial rates of pay were first established. Hence, unless their pay was increased it would be difficult for the asylum staff to maintain themselves. Hence, he proposed a new scale of payment (see Table 4.3).[99]

By 1860, wages of attendants in the asylum were less than what they would have earned in any other institution. Therefore, unless forced to do so from poverty or any dire necessity, attendants, according to the Surgeon of the Patna Lunatic Asylum, were unwilling to serve in the asylums. But as they were crucial for the management of the asylum and because it was difficult for the medical officers to function without their help, the Civil Surgeon of Patna, Dr Sutherland, proposed an increase in their salary. This, he thought, would ensure a 'respectable class of attendants' in the asylum, who would then be content to remain permanently in the institution.[100]

It was not only to retain the asylum staff at their posts, or to recruit a 'respectable class of attendants' that the medical officials argued in favour of increasing the pay but also because of the increase in the incident of

[98] Home, Public Proceedings, Medical, Bengal, Number 12, 27 April 1860, Letter sent from J. Sutherland, Civil Surgeon, Patna to H. D. H. Fergusson, Commissioner of Patna, letter dated 10 March 1860, APAC, BL.

[99] Home, Public Proceedings, Bengal, Number 12, Letter from J. Sutherland to H. D. H. Fergusson, 10 March 1860.

[100] Home, Public Proceedings, Bengal, Number 12, Letter from J. Sutherland to H. D. H. Fergusson, 10 March 1860.

Table 4.3 Present (1860) and Proposed Pay of the 'Native' Workers
of the Asylum

	Present Pay	
Number	Establishment	Total Amount in Rupees
1	Daroga	10
2	Jemadar at Rs 5 each	10
10	Keepers at Rs 3 each	30
4	Sweepers at Rs 3 each	12
1	Head Female Keeper	3
2	Female Keepers	6
1	Gardener	3
Total		74
	Proposed Pay	
Number	Establishment	Total Amount in Rupees
1	Daroga	20
1	Jemadar	10
	2nd Jemadar	8
10	Keepers at Rs 4 each	40
4	Sweepers at Rs 4 each	16
1	Head Female Keeper	5
2	Female Keepers at Rs 4 each	8
1	Gardener	4
Total		111

Source: Home Public Proceedings, Medical Department, Bengal, Number 12, 27
April, 1860, letter dated 10 March sent from J. Sutherland, Civil Surgeon, Patna to
H. D. H. Fergusson, Commissioner of Patna. APAC, BL.

thefts in the asylum, which they hinted the attendants were responsible
for. Officials at the Patna Lunatic Asylum complained about instances of
theft in the asylum, which they indicated was a consequence of low rates
of pay of the attendants. For instance, according to River Thomson, Junior
Secretary to the Government of Bengal, the 'wretched'[101] keepers, who

[101] Home, Public Proceedings, Medical, Bengal, Number 11, 27 April 1860,
Letter sent from H. D. H. Fergusson, Commissioner of Patna, to the Secretary
to the Government of Bengal, letter number 36, dated 2 April 1860, APAC, BL.

received a lower pay than was sufficient to support themselves and their families, had a great temptation to steal. Therefore, according to him, an increase in pay would help to control such a mischief in the asylum.

The Commissioner of Patna in 1860 forwarded the orders of the Lieutenant Governor the proposition submitted by the Civil Surgeon of Patna thereby soliciting an increase in the pay of the establishment at the Patna Asylum.[102] Under such circumstances, the Lieutenant Governor solicited the sanction of the Government of India for the additional expenditure proposed.[103] The government paid for the inmates in 'native' asylums but under these circumstances inmates became the victims of the situation. In the period between any proposal and its sanction, patients were always made to do extra labour. The profit procured from the sale of their manufactured products was used to pay the asylum staff.

The Lieutenant Governor was finally convinced that the monthly wages of keepers at the rate of Rs 4 was inadequate to secure trustworthy attendants and was, therefore prepared to move the higher quarters to sanction an increase of Rs 1 per month. He objected to the mutual dependency of the wages of the attendants on the profit of the labours of the inmates and pointed out that an increase in the pay should be compensated by the state.[104] In reality this was not practised.

The revised rules for the management of the Bengal asylums of 1860 finally sanctioned for one deputy keeper for every thirty patients, and one barkandaze or peon for every eight patients. One head female keeper was approved for female inmates and only one female coolie for eight female patients. No special night attendants were appointed. To compensate for the situation, barkandazes were supposed to divide the day and night duties amongst themselves. As this arrangement did not

[102] Home, Public Proceedings, Medical, Bengal, Number 11, Letter from H. D. H. Fergusson to Secretary to the Government of Bengal, 2 April 1860.

[103] Home, Public Proceedings, Medical, Bengal, Number 14, 27 April 1860, Letter sent to the Secretary to the Government of India from Rivers Thomson, Junior Secretary to the Government of Bengal, Home Department, letter number 181, dated 27 April 1860, APAC, BL.

[104] Home, Public Proceedings, Medical, Bengal, Number 5, 4 February 1862, Letter sent to the Principal Inspector General, Medical Department from Officiating Junior Secretary to the Government of Bengal, Letter number 22, dated 4 February 1862, APAC, BL.

solve the problem, by 1867, the government sanctioned, as a temporary measure, the employment of five extra keepers for night duties—four male and one female. The attendants were not permitted to sleep in the dormitories, but on the verandas close to the doors of the wards. Night guards were appointed to inspect inmates from cell to cell all through the night, and were punished if found asleep.[105] At the Bhawanipore Lunatic Asylum, attendants did not have the order to sleep in the wards unless it was convenient for them to do so.[106]

By the new regulations of 1860, paying patients admitted in the 'native' asylums were allowed to keep their private attendants. There were no separate rules for their payment as it depended on the employer personally and was not drawn from the government fund. For instance, in 1863, at Dullunda, those few patients who were admitted and had their maintenance paid for by their families, had the privilege of appointing private servants to look after them and to cook their meals.[107]

At the Moydapore Asylum, by October 1869, a mehtarnee was appointed because a new female ward was built. An extra barkandaze was also appointed in consequence of the increase in the total number of patients at the asylum.[108] By 1870, the overseer, Mr Frawley, was succeeded by a 'native' daroga on the proposal of the Deputy Inspector General of Hospitals at the cost of Rs 25 a month.[109]

In 1870, the system of shifts was introduced. Attendants were given hourly breaks in between their working hours. Henceforth, the head

[105] Home Department Proceedings, 19 December 19 1868, Letter from James Wise, Superintendent of the Lunatic Asylum, Dacca to William Keates, Deputy Inspector General of Hospitals, Dacca Circle, dated 24 June 1868, NAI.

[106] Home Department Proceedings, 19 December 1868, Letter sent to W. Keates, Deputy General of Hospitals, Presidency Circle from A. Payne, Superintendent of Asylum at the Presidency, Bhawanipore, dated 17 June 1868, NAI.

[107] A. Payne, 'Annual Report of the Dullunda Lunatic Asylum,' sent to H. M. Macpherson, 29 January 1863, *Annual Reports and Returns of the Insane Asylums in Bengal for the Years 1862–66.*

[108] John White, 'Report on Moydapore Asylum for 1869,' dated 18 January 1870, *Annual Report on the Insane Asylums in Bengal for the Year 1869.*

[109] Deputy Inspector General of Hospitals, G. Saunders's Report on the Moydapore Asylum, Enclosed to 'Report on Moydapore Asylum for 1869' by John White, NAI.

jemadar remained on duty from 5 AM to 8 PM. The other four jemadars were allowed only two and a half hours of break during the day for meals, and each one of them was allotted four hours of duty every night. The negabans in turn took breaks and went outside the asylum for two and half hours during the day, but at night all of them remained in the asylum and performed their duties alternately. The three hospital attendants were on duty all day except during their lunch breaks, and in their turn they had to work for an extra four hours at night. The average working hours of the attendant were fourteen hours in a day. They were employed in directing the work of the inmates, supervising that no quarrel broke out among them, preserving discipline and good behaviour, which included persuading the idle and refractory patients to obey the rules of the asylum, and treating the sick and 'demented' patients with kindness and consideration. To fulfil those duties properly, superintendent of the asylum felt the need for hiring a man with qualifications higher than that of *chowkeedars* or barkandazes.[110]

Also judging by the duration of their service, and their qualification, which he considered as inappropriate, the superintendent stated that their appointment in an asylum was temporary. For instance, out of the twenty-six male establishments in the Dacca Lunatic Asylum in 1871, only six keepers served over nine years, one less than five years, six keepers for less than three, and thirteen of them served for less than one year.[111]

According to Dr Wise, as wages of all kinds were rising rapidly, it was hopeless to expect any but the lowest class of men to accept service on a salary as insignificant as Rs 5 a month. He further stated that in Dacca, a coolie and a *rajmistry* (chief artisan) earned 5 *anna*s a day. The wages in asylums were low in comparison to those given by other departments to staff at similar positions. In jails, warders were paid Rs 6 a month. In the police force, the pay was higher than that in the asylum, the lowest grade constable received from Rs 5 to Rs 9 a month, and Rs 4 a year for clothing. In addition to these, a jail constable also gained rewards for seizure of smuggled opium and other contraband articles. Even a head constable

[110] Home, Public, Medical, Number 11, December 1871, Letter sent to the Deputy Inspector General of Hospitals, Dacca Circle, from Dr Wise, Superintendent of the Lunatic Asylum, Dacca, Number 176, dated 5 August 1871, NAI.

[111] Home, Public, Medical, Number 11, Letter from Dr Wise to the Deputy Inspector General of Hospitals, 5 August 1871.

earned Rs 25 a month, which gradually increased to Rs 60. This difference in pay was shown by the superintendent in order to point out the fact that the scale of pay prevalent in the asylum was unlikely to induce a respectable class of workers to accept employment in the asylum. Under such circumstances, he expected that a uniform rate of Rs 6 would improve the situation of the establishment. The superintendent stated that,

> in considering a revision of the scale if paid it should be borne in mind that government while establishing asylums had acknowledged the obligation of taking care of those unfortunate individuals who were bereft of reason, and of providing them with every reasonable requirement that would attract men was very judicious.[112]

The pay in the establishment was, therefore, determined by the local rate of wages, and, more specifically, by the pay that would induce 'Hindustanis'—a term used by the medical officials to refer to up-country men—to take up the job. Hindustanis were preferred for the work because of their physique and intelligence and their ability to work hard even in the 'uncongenial' climate of eastern Bengal. Although up-country men were appointed for the post of asylum staff as early as in the 1820s, by the late 1860s they were encouraged and preferred more than the local Bengalis by the medical officials. By 1860, at Dacca Asylum, four of the jemadars were residents of Dacca, and only one of Oudh. Of the attendants, nine belonged to Dacca, nine to Bihar, one to Mymensingh, one to Allahabad, and one to Madras, illustrating that there were more local men involved in it than from other states, but the medical officers demanded for a change.[113]

The superintendent, after consulting those best acquainted with eastern Bengal, arrived at the conclusion that a salary of Rs 6 would induce men to take permanent employment in Bengal. Therefore, he proposed that the scale of pay should be graduated, and that the jemadars should receive a salary that would entitle them to the benefits of the pension rules as well. Under this scheme, it was decided that five senior negabans after serving for five years would receive Rs 7, while the rest of them

[112] Home, Public, Medical, Number 11, Letter from Dr Wise to the Deputy Inspector General of Hospitals, 5 August 1871.

[113] Home, Public, Medical, Number 11, Letter from Dr Wise to the Deputy Inspector General of Hospitals, 5 August 1871.

would get Rs 6 a month.[114] An increase in pay not only drew more attendants to such work but it also allowed the space for implementing stricter discipline and supervision of the asylum staff.

Amongst the asylum staff, the attendants, because of their officious engagement with the inmates, were also held responsible for patients escaping from the asylum. In such circumstances, a minor quibble was considered insufficient to punish the attendants. Therefore, according to the Superintendent of the Dacca Asylum, the government needed to make asylum attendants liable for the same punishment as jail barkandazes for allowing prisoners to escape, and that Section 223 of the Indian Penal Code, and Section 2 of Act IV of 1867 needed to be enforced within asylums as it was within jails. This Act was particularly meant to punish male attendants whereas female attendants were kept outside its jurisdiction. This was because of the difficulties in engaging the latter in work depended on causes other than those mentioned in the case of men. According to the superintendent, the majority of women who were recruited as attendants were elderly Muslim widows, who were usually left with other dependents on them. As young women were not appointed for the post of attendants, he did not want to discharge those who were already appointed. He wanted to increase their pay to retain them in the service longer.

Of the seven women working at Dullunda, three women had served over three years, and the remaining women served for two years. Other than working at the asylum the only service those women pursued outside the asylum was that of dhais with Armenian or Muslim families where they were paid Rs 3 a month including food and clothing. The scarcity of women workers as attendants made the superintendent anxious. Therefore, he recommended an increase in the pay of the female asylum staffs, which was as follows: the *jemadarny* was to be paid Rs 8, the two senior negabans, if employed for over five years would receive Rs 6 each, and the remaining female attendants were to be continued at a salary of Rs 5 each. As a result of this, the total increase in pay was Rs 9 per month.[115] Female attendants were needed as much as male

[114] Home, Public, Medical, Number 11, Letter from Dr Wise to the Deputy Inspector General of Hospitals, 5 August 1871.

[115] Home, Public, Medical, Number 11, Letter from Dr Wise to the Deputy Inspector General of Hospitals, 5 August 1871.

attendants, but in the absence of their easy availability, rules were relaxed in case of the former.

Strict rules were also imposed regarding the duties of the asylum staff along with an increase in their pay. Unlike in the 1860s, when only fines were imposed for negligence, by the 1870s they were suspended on similar grounds. For instance, at the Patna Asylum in 1872, three keepers were dismissed with forfeiture of all pay for ill-treating inmates under their charge. At the same time, the number of keepers was increased and they were also paid higher salaries than before.[116] In another instance, according to a local newspaper of Moorshedabad, a 'lunatic' patient had escaped from the Moorshedabad Asylum on the day of the marriage of the daroga's daughter. The Magistrate of Moorshedabad and the inspectors of the asylum were asked to enquire into the matter, and to let the public know the result of their enquiries. This showed that not only was the daroga held responsible for the matter, but at the end of the nineteenth century, asylum officials were also answerable to the public regarding their conduct.[117]

Of the eight attendants at Cuttack Asylum, one was a supernumerary, sanctioned for a temporary period, but by 1872, the average number of lunatics was over fifty, and two of the attendants were women. Along with this, the Superintendent Surgeon thought it necessary to appoint an extra warder. This was necessary because five keepers were not enough to look after forty male inmates, given that they had to perform both day and night duties, in comparison to two women attendants in charge of ten female patients. The keepers were paid the same rate of Rs 6 per head monthly. The Superintendent Surgeon believed that an increase of Rs 2 would improve the situation further. He, therefore, proposed to increase the rate by Rs 2 for one keeper and Rs 1 for another, thereby making the pay of one keeper Rs 8 and another Rs 7. He proposed a reward for the best attendant, to motivate them to work harder in a service where the duties were both arduous and responsible.[118] Such rewards were given as an incentive not only to make them permanent in the establishment

---

[116] B. Simpson, 'Report on the Patna Lunatic Asylum for the Year ending 31 December 1872,' *Annual Report on the Insane Asylums of Bengal for the Year 1872.*

[117] *Murshidabad Hitaishi*, 16 May 1894, NAI.

[118] H. Cayley, 'Report on the Cuttack Lunatic Asylum for the Year 1872,' H. Cayley, *Annual Report on the Insane Asylums of Bengal for the Year 1872.*

but also to encourage them in their duties. This kind of sub-divisions of the post also continued in practice like it happened at Patna Asylum as mentioned earlier.

The average cost of establishment varied from one asylum to the other. For instance, the excess in establishment charges, at Dullunda and Dacca, which the Superintendent Surgeon of Asylums of Bengal thought proper, was due to the higher rates of wages ruling at those places. Except in the wages of sweepers, there was little difference between the rates of the establishment at Patna and those at Dacca.[119] This circumstance, however, did not altogether explain the excess. Reference was made in previous resolutions to the inequalities in the strength of establishment at different asylums. The excess cost at Dacca was due to undue multiplication of paid attendants rather than high wages.

In 1886, the Medico Psychological Association, the organization of asylum doctors, published the *Handbook for the Instruction of Attendants on the Insane*,[120] in which they stated that the remuneration and privileges of efficient attendants should be as liberal as possible and any special aptitude for work should receive recognition and reward. Although there was an attempt in the asylums of Bengal to provide the asylum staff with a proper scale of pay and to give them rewards for their maintenance and care of the patients, the situation did not improve. The issue of the pay of attendants remained problematic and subject to constant change throughout the nineteenth century.

'RESTRAINT' PRACTISED BY THE ASYLUM STAFF

The asylum staff members were supposed to manage the inmates without using any kind of restraints. They were expected not to be harsh or use any kind of physical coercion while treating patients. Robert Gardiner Hill, Member of the Royal College of Surgeons, in a lecture

[119] Bengal Home, Medical Proceedings, Number 9, May 1881, Resolution Medical and Municipal Department, Medical, Calcutta, dated 25 May 1881, APAC, BL.

[120] Medico Psychological Association, *Handbook for the Instruction of Attendants on the Insane* (Boston: Cupples, Upham and Company, 1886), 136, WL.

delivered on the abolition of mechanical restraint, stated that an alternative to mechanical restraint included classification and watchfulness, vigilant and unceasing attendance. It also included kindness, occupation, and attention to health, cleanliness, and comfort of inmates. He further stated that in an asylum there should be a sufficient number of strong, tall, and active attendants, whose remuneration must be such as to secure persons of good character, and steady principle, to undertake their arduous duties.[121]

To prevent any kind of corporal punishment at the Dacca Lunatic Asylum, the attendants were not allowed to carry sticks or canes or any other sharp objects.[122] According to Daniel Tuke:

> It must not be forgotten that one of the first objects in view, in placing a patient in an asylum, is security, by which is implied that he shall be secure from individual harm, and that the community shall be secure from receiving injury from him.[123]

A man was sent to the Patna Lunatic Asylum from the Santhal district of the Lower Provinces of Bengal. He was ferocious, and had a propensity to seize anyone who came near him and bite them severely. His treatment was a trial of the system of non-restraint. A keeper was separately appointed for him. This showed good results, as he gradually yielded to the treatment of the keeper, and in a few weeks, became quiet and orderly. The Deputy Inspector General of Hospitals exalted the greater attention on the part of the keepers.[124] Prior to the practice of non-restraint, this man would have been locked up but the new mode of treatment and care of

---

[121] Robert Gardiner Hill, *A Concise History of the Entire Abolition of Mechanical Restraint in the Treatment of the Insane; and of the Introduction, Success, and Final Triumph of the Non Restraint System, Together with a Reprint of a Lecture Delivered on the Subject in the Year 1838 and Appendices, Containing an Account of the Controversies and Claims Connected Therewith* (London: Longman, Brown, Green, and Longmans, Paternoster Row, 1857), WL.

[122] Medical Board Proceedings, Letter from J. Taylor to Robert Brown, 2 May 1842.

[123] Tuke, *Moral Management of the Insane*, 115.

[124] Home Public Department, Medical Board Proceedings, Number 43, dated 27 February 1862, Letter number 134, dated 18 February 1862, sent to E. H. Lushington, Secretary to the Government of Bengal, from J. Forsyth, Principal Inspector General, Medical Department, APAC, BL

inmates made a difference. The superintendent particularly noted that the category of 'ferocious maniacs' had disappeared.[125] Therefore, no patient was locked up during the year in the daytime. This he attributed chiefly to the employment of inmates, which provided an outlet for superfluous energy; but he also believed that it was partly dependant on the proper carrying out of the non-restraint system.

According to the Inspector General of Hospitals of Bengal Presidency, adoption of restraint in all the asylums inculcated and maintained among attendants an entirely false and wrong notion as to how inmates should be treated. It was impossible to dissociate, except in the surgical cases, the idea of coercion or punishment from the imposition of restraint.[126] He further stated that such an idea was prone to govern all the details of an institution in which restraint was a recognized element in the management of 'mad' people. The imposition of manual restraint was by no means a necessary alternative, and was seldom found requisite in asylums where the idea and practice of restraint was abolished.[127]

According to John Conolly,

an indispensable condition for protecting and controlling the insane, without having recourse to bodily restraints, is the command of the services of a sufficient number of efficient attendants.[128]

Although a desirable situation, it was difficult to implement such ideas into practice because many factors were related to a proper functioning of the asylum establishment.

The issue of pay, the asylum staffs' care towards inmates, their sense of duty and responsibilities, all continued to be important throughout

[125] Home Public Department, Medical Board Proceedings, Number 43, Letter number 134 from J. Forsyth to E. H. Lushington, dated 18 February 1862.

[126] Home, Public, Medical, Bengal, Number 21, 4 October 1872, Letter sent to the Officiating Secretary to the Government of Bengal from J. Campbell Brown, Inspector General of Hospitals, Indian Medical Department, on the Report of the Asylums of Bengal, Fort William, dated 27 June 1872, APAC, BL.

[127] Home, Public, Medical, Bengal, Number 21, Letter from J. Campbell Brown to Officiating Secretary to the Government of Bengal, 27 June 1872.

[128] Conolly, *The Construction and Government of Lunatic Asylums and Hospitals*, 83.

the nineteenth century. Problems increased over time with an increase in the number of attendants of the establishment along with the growing number of asylums. This entire issue over pay was initiated by the medical officers who depended on the asylum staff for the maintenance and care of inmates. They tried to increase the pay on several instances to sustain the staff in the asylum. After all, the officers had to engage themselves in practising new theories on insanity rather than looking after the daily care and maintenance of patients. The medical officers then increasingly depended on the asylum staff for their duties. This resulted in a shift. The asylum staff got more involved with the inmates than the medical officers. While medical officers initially took the decisions concerning the patients, gradually the asylum staff took over the role of decision-making.

The asylum staff represented the inmates in an asylum. The superintendent of an asylum who was to visit it regularly was gradually absent from his duties by the middle of the nineteenth century because his duties were gradually replaced by the presence of the asylum staff. Therefore, the contact hours between the superintendents and inmates slowly reduced and there was no direct interaction between the two any more. Instead, the asylum staff acted as a mediator. According to Andrew Scull, it broke the tie between the patient and the physician, which the proponents of the asylum had believed to be an important feature of asylum life.[129] The asylum staff was appointed to replace the practice of mechanical restraint in the asylum, although how far that actually worked remained doubtful. There were instances when attendants mismanaged the inmates and were dismissed from their jobs. But the question remained that if mechanical restraint had to be replaced by the role of attendants, then why were attendants not trained accordingly, which was extremely necessary for the successful functioning of the post. Throughout the nineteenth century, no such attempts were ever made. Therefore, a gap existed between 'rhetoric and reality'[130] in understanding the role of attendants.

Within the closed walls of the asylum, the staff taught inmates to be disciplined and humane by engaging and supervising them in various activities so that they could lead a civilized social life once they were

[129] Scull, *The Most Solitary of Afflictions*, 172.

[130] For further discussion on the issue, see Anne Digby, *Madness, Mortality and Medicine: A Study of the York Retreat, 1796-1914* (Cambridge: Cambridge University Press, 1985), 140–69.

released. Their duty involved an officious intrusion into the personal space of the patient. They were usually appointed all through day and night for the constant surveillance on the inmates without any leave, until the 1870s when a system of shifts and standardized duty hours were allotted for them, whereby they were allowed to take regular breaks. It improved the position of the asylum staff to a great extent.

This relationship between the asylum staff and the patient was symbiotic—any harm caused to one affected the other. On the other hand, attendants' reports on inmates determined their modes of treatment and duration of stay in an asylum, as well as their supply of sweetmeats, tobacco, and other incentives. At the same time, an attendant who was found to be rude or harsh to any patient was dismissed from his job. However, the ultimate power lay in the hands of the asylum staff and therefore, the fact that they were in a vantage position to care for or to discriminate against the patients was also true.

CONCLUSION

THIS BOOK IS AN IN-DEPTH study of the asylums of Bengal, along with the various definitions of insanity, geographical and environmental reasons behind the choice of location of asylums, and different methods of treatment practised within their walls. Even with the construction of new asylums or an expansion of the existing structures, the asylum authorities failed to control the increase in admission of patients, not necessarily because different types of insanity were on an increase, but because the asylum administrators found it difficult to provide accommodation for them. Repeated cases of readmission and over-lapping of different categories of mental illnesses further complicated the situation. It worsened when more inmates were admitted into the asylums, which not only included new cases, but also readmissions of previously cured and discharged patients who suffered relapses. Medical officers were worried under such circumstances as asylums did not have enough space to accommodate patients. Also, the treatment of many cases got delayed because of the layers of the disease, ranging from suicidal melancholy to physical symptoms such as dysentery. All these problems over-burdened the asylum infrastructure. This resulted in medical officers hastily treating patients to discharge them from asylums. This in turn left the problem unresolved and the treatment incomplete. This again led to a proportionate increase in cases of readmission. By the end of the nineteenth century, there were discussions for the construction of a central lunatic asylum, which the medical officers thought would not only help to solve the problem but also to manage the situation.

Inside the asylum, patients underwent painful experiences for various reasons. For example, an important cause of difficulty that was particularly faced by the inmates of the European Lunatic Asylum was that on failing to make necessary arrangements for payment for their maintenance, they were usually shifted from the first-class category to the second. As notions of class and race determined the social life of Victorian England, for European patients, a shift in their position even within the asylum was detrimental to their class status and pride. In the 'native' asylums where most of the patients belonged to the lower class, the situation was different. Inmates were transferred from one asylum to another because of lack of space and provisions. This further increased their mental and physical stress. Most of the patients were physically and mentally weak when they were initially admitted to asylums, their journeys to distant asylums further worsened their health. Additionally, police and attendants were recorded to have 'mishandled' them en route. Therefore, many of them died soon after their transfer from one asylum to the other. The inmates, therefore, faced traumatic experiences not only after their admission, but even before they were admitted to the asylums. The stringent therapeutic regime further worsened their health. Hence, many inmates attempted to escape from the asylums.

By the mid-nineteenth century, moral treatment gained significance, and accordingly the inner and outer design of the buildings were also changing. The construction of an asylum varied according to the site, environment, geographical location, and transport facilities including waterways, and this entire process was determined by varying inter-pretations of the disease. The types and numbers of wards and rooms constructed not only depended on how the medical officers categorized insanity—between violent and non-violent forms, and the total number of inmates admitted in an asylum—but it was also determined by methods of treatment practised. The construction of solitary cells also became a necessary part of asylum construction as an aspect of moral therapy.

An important issue determining the choice of location was the availability of dry and well-ventilated sites. The medical officers emphasized the importance of construction on a high and dry land, as wet, swampy, and marshy lands often delayed the recovery of patients. The engineers constructing asylums designed the inner wards, rooms, and verandas overlooking open courtyards. Therefore, the construction of an asylum and the spatial distribution within it was related to the question of treatment, which in turn reflected understandings of insanity.

The methods of treatment at asylums and the knowledge of mental illness among medical practitioners in nineteenth-century India were sites of exchange and solely derivative.

During the early nineteenth century, asylums were initially set up in India to remove the 'abnormal' and the 'deviants' from civilized society and confine them in a separate place away from the town or city. This peripheral location showed that insanity was not considered as a disease but as a cause of shame for colonial society. Insanity, considered untreatable, led to the establishment of asylums as sites of shame, hidden away at the margins of the town. Towards the end of the nineteenth century, the location of asylums and the interpretations of madness as a disease were changing. Asylum buildings began to be constructed within the boundaries of a town or city. This showed that insanity was beginning to be considered as a medically curable disease. Towards the latter half of the nineteenth century, the moral aspect of insanity lost its value while the medical aspect increasingly gained dominance: moral treatment was gradually replaced and increasingly dominated by medical treatment towards the end of the nineteenth century, when insanity began to be recognized as a curable disease.

Usually, the medical practitioners placed in asylums were not par-ticularly trained in treating mental illness. These physicians dealt with general illnesses, most of them were not trained to treat mental diseases. In fact, the definitions and classifications of insanity varied from one asylum to another. After several exchanges of ideas amongst medical practitioners in Bengal, a generalized treatment of insanity began to be practised. General bodily diseases were separately dealt with; these ranged from general weakness of the body to the treatment of several symptomatic diseases.

Prior case histories of patients were recorded in a book, *Descriptive Rolls*, upon admission. It was a register that maintained the detailed report of the past records of every inmate except those whose previous history remained unknown. This record was either based on the observations of a physician outside the asylum whom the patient first visited or on the observation of family members, friends, or acquaintances. The asylum physicians found it difficult to deal with those cases that did not have a prior case history, and they often left those cases untreated. This illustrated that by knowing the previous case history, they tried to understand the type of insanity, and thereby classified them accordingly inside the asylums, while it also showed that they were unable to address new case histories of which they had no prior knowledge and necessary training. Therefore, the patients who failed to register a prior case history were categorized as 'unknown'.

Until the nineteenth century, the definition of insanity was fluid; the situation became complicated when medical officers tried to formulate the causes of female insanity as different from that of males. This was understood differently not because of the biological differences between men and women. The difference should be perceived as a social construction, which looked at women as not only weak, but also emotional. Thus, their emotional exuberances, the medical officers thought, often led to an imbalance in their expressions, which made them laugh, cry, sing, or talk to themselves. They considered the menstrual cycle as an important factor in understanding women's insanity. Therefore, her sanity was related to the regular flow of her menses. Hence, the treatment of a female patient was different from that of a male patient.

In the process of treatment, European physicians took help of the 'natives' whom they considered ignorant, but whom they could also not ignore entirely; for instance, the appointment of 'native' doctors, 'native' attendants, and also 'native' patients in the day-to-day functioning of the asylums. The role of the asylum staff members became significant as mechanical treatment was gradually replaced by moral treatment and also as more asylums were built and more patients admitted into them. Eventually, for the daily maintainance and care of inmates, the role of the physicians was replaced by the asylum staff members. The latter not only had the power to take decisions in situations of crisis, but were also in charge of providing the patients with medicines prescribed by the doctors. They were responsible for their care and treatment, and had a mutual relationship with them. This was supposed to improve the condition of inmates, but over time it led to another set of problems as the attendants were not medically trained.

The asylum physicians established an understanding of insanity, which eventually emerged as a special field of discipline, known as psychiatry, towards the beginning of twentieth century. This was not only about mental health, but about the whole range of medical activities that they were engaged in, which increasingly dominated the colonial asylum system.

Asylums and life within those institutions in the twenty-first century, hence, is a continuation of how it existed in the nineteenth century and continued to be so even in the twentieth century. Categories changed over time as Insane Hospitals or Lunatic Asylums began to be called 'Mental Hospital', 'Institute of Psychiatry', or 'Institute of Psychiatry and Behavioural Sciences', but nothing much changed beyond this. Although the government began addressing the issue of mental illness to increase awareness among the people from the end of the twentieth century until the present day, places of confinement are still found in a hopeless condition where the disorderly mind continues to exist in its own world of orderliness, oblivious to the world outside.

APPENDICES

APPENDIX I: RULES PROPOSED FOR THE CONTROL AND MANAGEMENT OF THE EUROPEAN INSANE HOSPITAL[1]

Control and Superintendence

1. The general control and superintendence of the hospital for European Insane at this presidency is vested in the medical board and in the magistrates of Calcutta.

2. The first member of the medical board and the principal magistrate of Calcutta shall visit the hospital together on the first day of every month; and in those visits they well inspect minutely and make particular enquiries into the state of each patient. They will on the 1st day of each month also submit to the govt a return of the patients in the hospital signed by them conjointly. With this return they well furnish a report containing their sentiments on the general state of the hospital; and on its management in so far as regards the comfort and welfare of the patients, with reference to food, clothing, cleanliness, medical treatment and humane care and attention on the part of the Surgeon of the hospitals and those employed under his authority.

3. Any of the magistrate of Calcutta shall visit the hospital as often as they may think it necessary. It will be the duty of the several members of the

[1] Medical Board Proceedings, Number 38, 28 November 1817, Enclosure attached to a Letter sent to Mr Trotter, Secretary to Government in Public Department from R. Leny, Secretary Medical Board, dated 6 November 1817, NAI.

Medical Board to visit it frequently; and to control and direct the general management and professional treatment of the patients. They will be held responsible that due care and attention is bestowed upon the patients in every respect and that no deficiency is permitted in regard to any object that may be conducive either to the welfare and comfort of their unhappy situation or to their ultimate recovery.

4. It is the intention of Government that a Surgeon and an Assistant Surgeon shall be appointed for the immediate charge and management of the insane hospital, under the control and direction above mentioned. It is also intended that those gentlemen shall constantly reside either at or near the immediate vicinity of the hospital; and in order to ensure their whole time and attention being exclusively devoted to the care of the patient that they shall hold in other situation not appointment, and that they shall abstain from all private practice except when called to visit persons afflicted with insanity and from every other pursuit which can interfere in the most remote degree with the care and proper conduct of the establishment committed to their charge.

5. Persons belonging to any of the corps of the army who are afflicted with derangement shall be sent to the insane hospital after having been examined and reported to be insane by a medical committee to be assembled for that purpose. Persons in the civil and marine departments will be admitted into the hospital after their insanity has been certified in respect to civil servants by two medical practitioners in Calcutta and in respect to marine servants; by the marine surgeon and his assistant. The insanity of persons unconnected with the public service shall in all practicable cases be certified by two medical practitioners before they are admitted into the hospital. The reports of medical committee in cases of insanity in the military department and the certificates in all the other several instances above mentioned are to be transmitted to the surgeon of the hospital by whom they are to be carefully preserved. Transcripts of these reports and certificates are in every case to be made in a Book of records which is to be kept at the hospital for that purpose; and the authenticity of those copies is to be certified by the signature of the Surgeon of the Hospital.

6. All patients admitted into the hospital shall be visited and examined by the senior member of the medical Board immediately on their admission or as soon afterwards as possible. That officer shall furnish the surgeon of the hospital with his opinion in writing respecting the person admitted with reference to the state of the malady and the propriety of the future detention of the patients. The writing containing this opinion is to be carefully preserved by the Surgeon of the Hospital and a transcript of it is to be made in the Book of Records above mentioned immediately

subjoined to the report or certificate relating to the same patient. The authenticity of this copy is likewise to be certified by the signature of the surgeon of the hospital.

7. Patients shall be discharged from the hospital only by the authority of the visiting member of the medical board in ordinary cases; and in every instance when a patient is discharge that officer will furnish the surgeon of the Hospital with his opinion in writing in respect to the propriety and safety of the discharge. This writing like those above mentioned will be carefully preserved; and it shall be transcribed under a distinct head for patients discharged in the Board of Record which has been already discharged. This transcript shall likewise be authenticated in every instance by the signature of the surgeon of the hospital. The senior member of the medical board and the principal magistrate of Calcutta in all their monthly visits to the hospital shall carefully inspect this Book of Record and in their reports to the Government shall state whether the above directions are duly and regularly compiled with by the medical officer having the immediate charge of the hospital.

8. Besides this record it will be the duty of the surgeon of the hospital to keep a separate book in which the case of each patient is to be particularly described; and the name, period of admission, age, country, temperament, pursuits and habits of the patient and the history of the disease so far as it may be possible to ascertain those circumstances carefully detailed. The medical treatment and general management of each patient shall also time to time be described in this Book, together with the success attending the measures adopted for the cure of the patient. In cases of bodily indisposition a daily report of the disease and its treatment shall be entered in this book and the event whether in death or recovery stated as is usual in ordinary medical journals. The progressive result of the treatment for the cure of insanity, the periods of the disease of patients or in cases of recovery those of their discharge shall also be carefully recorded. This Book shall be attentively inspected in the periodical visits of the senior member of the medical board and the principal magistrate of Calcutta who in their reports to the govt will state whether this record is duly and regularly kept by the surgeon of the hospital.

9. Both the Surgeon of the Hospital and his Assistant shall regularly visit the hospital in the morning and again in the evening of each day; and they shall at every visit carefully inspect the case of each patient in the hospital; and adopt such measures as may appear necessary under the particular circumstances that shall from time to time occur. Besides these stated visits the Surgeon and his Assistant shall at all other times give their attendance in the hospital when required by the situation of any patient. In this manner

due care and attention are to be extended generally to the duties of the hospital; and particularly to the separate case of every patient under all its peculiar circumstances and variations.

10. The Surgeon of the Hospital shall furnish to the Medical Board a weekly return of his patients prepared according to the form above laid down for that which is to be submitted monthly to the govt.; and it shall be accompanied by a report of all circumstances requiring the Boards notice in any of the branches of that establishment. The surgeon shall also furnish to the Adjutant General of the army for the information of His Excellency the Commander in Chief, a quarterly return and report of all patients belonging to the military department who are in the hospital. This return will also be prepared according to the form above specified.

Supply to the Hospital

1. The diet, clothing, bedding and all necessaries for the patients in the insane hospital with the exception of medicines and surgical instruments shall be supplied by the Department of the Commissariat. This mode of supply shall commence on the 1st of January 1818 previously to which time the Commissariat shall receive from the Surgeon at present in charge of that establishment all hospital stores belonging to him at such rates as may be adjudged proper by the senior member of the medical board and an officer of the Commissariat after having conjointly examined and appreciated the value of the stores in question.

2. The articles of clothing and bedding for the use of the patients in the hospital shall be of two different descriptions of which one shall be suitable for persons belonging to the higher and the other for persons of the lower rank of life. The clothing and the bedding generally shall be of the kind used by persons belonging to those ranks respectively when in health. Articles of this nature will be provided in sufficient quantity to afford to patients of the inferior class a change every second day of articles requiring to be washed, articles which do not require to be washed shall be changed and renewed only according to the judgement of the Surgeon of the Hospital confirmed by the visiting Member of the Medical Board.

3. When supplies of clothing, bedding, etc. are required for the use of the insane hospital an indent shall be prepared by the Surgeon of that establishment in which the number and description of the several articles required are particularly specified. This indent having been sanctioned by the signature of the visiting member of the medical board shall be complied with by the commissariat. On the delivery to the Surgeon of the hospital by the Commissariat of the articles required the Surgeon shall write a receipt on

the back of the indent which shall serve as a voucher to the commissariat for the supply which may have been provided.

4. The Commissariat shall in communication with the Medical Board prepare two sits of all the most important articles of clothing and bedding required for the two descriptions of patients whether male or female in the insane hospital. Every article of those sits [*sic*] when approved by the medical board shall have the seal of that office affixed to it. One of those sits shall be lodged with the Commissariat to guide that department in providing all supplies for the use of the hospital of the articles in question. The other sit shall be lodged among the stores of the insane hospital to serve as a standard for the kind and quality of articles to be here after furnished which the medical officers of that establishment may refer to whenever he may be of opinion that the clothing and bedding furnished are not of the description which is intended.

5. The diet of the patients in the insane hospital shall likewise be of two different descriptions according as the persons for whom it is intended shall belong to the higher or inferior class of patients. The diet for each class shall be generally of a description approximating to that used in ordinary circumstances by persons in health who belong to those classes respectively. It will however be of course subject to such regulation and modification at all times as may be proper and expedient in the judgement of the medical officers under whose guidance and direction the hospital is placed.

6. As the adoption of precise rules in respect to the diet of the patients in the insane hospital would not appear to be practicable the quality and quantity of all articles of diet furnished must be regulated by the judgement and description of the surgeon of that establishment acting under the control and superintendence of the medical board. The general supply of the several articles of diet to be furnished daily will be specified by the Surgeon of the Hospital to the Commissariat; and timely notice will be given to that department when variation in that supply are considered necessary or new or extra articles are required. The steward of the hospital shall grant to the agent employed by the Commissariat, a daily receipt countersigned by the Surgeon for all articles which the agent shall furnish at the end of every month a general list of all the articles of diet received from the commissariat during the month shall be prepared and signed by the Surgeon of the Hospital; and it shall afterwards be submitted to the visiting member of the medical board for his sanction; and when approved shall be signed by that officer and delivered to the commissariat. This list will be compared by that department with the daily receipts received by its agent from the steward of the hospital as above directed and will serve as a monthly voucher for the whole of the articles of diet furnished. By being subjected to the inspection

and by its requiring the sanction of the visiting member of the medical board it will at the same time enable that officer to judge generally of the supply furnished; and it will be his duty to interfere his authority when he may be of opinion that the supple of diet to the patients is conducted on a scale that is either in judicious and wasteful on the one hand or in any respect narrow and defective on the other.

7.   The wine with which it may be considered proper to supply any of the patients in the insane hospital shall in general be madiera wine of the same description with that used in the several hospitals for Europeans under this Presidency. Beer or other liquors however which are deemed necessary by the surgeon of the hospital for particular patients shall likewise be allowed all supplies of wine and articles of that description shall be furnished on indent presented to the Commissariat by the Surgeon of the hospital and bearing the countersignature of the senior member of the medical board. Monthly statements shall be submitted to that Board by the Surgeon of the hospital of the quantity of wine, and the articles of that description expended in the hospital. In these statements will be specified the reasons for which such articles are allowed, together with the quantity given to the several patients by whom they are used and it will be the duty of the visiting member of the medical board from time to time to compare these statements with the record kept by the surgeon of the hospital in his book of cases where the quantity of wine and etc. Granted to each patient and the circumstances requiring their use are to be carefully inserted.

8.   One or more weekly newspapers as the Surgeon of the hospital may think advisable will be allowed for the amusement of the patients in the insane hospital. Particular patients may also when it is deemed proper be supplied with books from the circulating libraries of Calcutta; and any other little indulgence which the surgeon may deem very expedient in certain cases shall be allowed. The Commissariat will therefore comply with requisitions made by the Surgeon of the hospital for articles of this description provided that in every case the requisition shall be countersigned by the visiting member of the medical board in testimony of the sanction and approbation of that controlling authority. It is the intention of the govt generally that no article which the medical board may think necessary, expedient or useful for any of the unhappy persons compered [sic] in the insane hospital shall be withheld, although they expected due attention to economy and moderation in respect to every supply that may be required.

9.   The cots, tables, chairs, &etc. Required for the insane hospital shall of the description which the medical board may think best suited for that establishment. These together with cooking, utensils, plates, table cloths, napkins, and every article of that description, shall be supplied by the

commissariat on indents prepared by the surgeon of the hospital and countersigned by the visiting member of the medical board. The hospital shall also be lighted up at night by the Commissariat, in the mode which the surgeon of the hospital, with the sanction of the medical board may think most proper. It shall also be the duty of the commissariat to preserve the walks and drains around the hospital and the whole of the space comprehended within or adjoining to the outside of the general enclosure wall free from weeds or soil of any description, and in a state of the greatest practicable cleanliness.

10. All the Europe and country medicine, surgical instruments and apothecary's, utensils which are required for the use of the insane hospital shall be supplied from the Honourable Company's Dispensary. Indents for such articles shall be prepared by the Surgeon of the hospital according to the form prescribed by the general medical regulations for the other hospitals under this presidency. These indents shall be submitted to the medical board by whom they will be examined and passed in the usual manner previously to their being complied with.

Charges for Patients in the Hospital

1. The allowance of all persons receiving pay from the Honourable Company will cease on their being admitted into the insane hospital as patients. To ensure the execution of this rule, it will be the duty of the surgeon of the hospital to notify the periods of admission and discharge of every patient, belonging to the military department to the military auditor general; and of every patient from the civil or marine departments to the civil auditor of account. Those officers guided by such notifications shall adopt the necessary measures for checking the issue of pay in their respective departments on account of public servants whose unhappy situations may have required their transference to the insane hospital.

2. The families of the persons referred to in the preceding paragraph to whim the arrangement above specified may be productive of circumstances of hardship and who may require support, will be pleased to make their situations and claims known to the govt through the medical board. It will be the duty of that board to submit to the govt all representations of this kind that may be presented to them; and they will at the same time furnish such further information in regard to each particular case, as they may be enabled to obtain, together with such observations as they may deem necessary. The govt in every case of this kind which is regularly brought before them will carefully consider the circumstances stated, and pass such orders as they may deem necessary or expedient in each particular instance.

3. Persons unconnected with the public service who may become patients in the insane hospital, will be maintained in that establishment from the proceeds of their own property, when their circumstances are adequate to that object, when the property of patients of this description is insufficient to defray their expenses in the insane hospital, it is reasonable and proper that these should become a charge on their relations and friends in all practicable cases. It will therefore be expected that the natural duty of maintaining persons in this unhappy situation will be undertaken by their connections who may possess the means of affording it.

4. The charges to be made in the cases referred to in the preceding paragraph will be at the rate of Rs. 100 per mensem for all patients belonging to the superior class, and of Rs. 30 per mensem for patients of the inferior class. These sums shall be collected by the Commissariat and credit given for them to the govt in the accounts of expenditure by that department, an account of the insane hospital. It will be required that sufficient security for the payment of the charges above mentioned shall accompany applications for the admission of patients of this description into the hospital; and these securities shall be preserved by the surgeon of the hospital for the purpose of being available when necessary by the commissariat. It will also be the duty of the surgeon of the hospital to transmit on the first day of every month a list of the names of all such patients in which are specified the class to which each belongs together with the periods of admission and discharge for the information and guidance of the military auditor general.

5. In all cases where it shall clearly appear that neither the friends of insane patients nor the circumstances of their relations and friends are adequate to defray the charges an account of their cure and maintenance in the insane hospital the necessary expenses on that account will be charged to the govt. Such patients on their admission into the hospital shall belong to the superior or inferior class of patients, according to the station and rank in life which they may have previously occupied.

6. In order that no expense but what is absolutely necessary may be incurred by the govt on account of patient received into the insane hospital, it will be the duty of the medical board to institute particular enquiries in respect to the circumstances of all patients admitted into that establishment for whom public support is required. These enquiries shall likewise extend to the situation and circumstance of the relations and friends of the insane persons. Such information as may be this procured shall be submitted to the govt in order that a correct judgement may be formed whether charitable consideration and support are necessary and proper. The orders which the govt may deem necessary in every particular case of this kind will be communicated to the medical board.

Servants of the Hospital

1. There shall be an European Steward and Apothecary in one person, who shall reside at the hospital and discharge his duties under the immediate direction and control of the surgeon of the hospital and his assistant. This person shall be furnished with quarters and receive a salary of Rs. 120 per month. There shall be two European male keepers, one of them for the superior and the other for the inferior class of patients. There shall also be a European female keeper for the female patients. These three persons shall discharge their duties under the immediate direction and control if the surgeon of the hospital and his assistant and a salary of Rs. 80 per month shall be granted to each of them together with quarters at the hospital.

2. There shall be one head 'native' male keeper for the superior class; and there shall be a head 'native' female keeper for the female patients the wages of each of these three persons shall be Rs. 12 per mensem. There shall be one ordinary 'native' male keeper for every two male patients and one ordinary 'native' female keeper for every two female patients. These persons shall each receive Rs. 8 per month as wages.

3. There shall be one metre for every four patients on the male department; and one materany for every similar number of patients in the female department; each of whom shall be allowed wages at the rate of Rs. 5 per month. Besides these there shall be one head metre, and one head materany at Rs. 6 per month each four Bullach [*sic*] bhesties shall be allowed for the general service of the hospital at Rs. 10 per month, each. There shall also be one head tailor and four ordinary tailors, the former at Rs. 8; and the latter at Rs. 7 per month each; together with one sircar [*sic*] or native water [*sic*] with a monthly allowance of Rs. 32.

4. Besides the fixed establishment of servants above mentioned the commissariat in communication with the surgeon of the hospital and the medical board will provide the requisite number of cooks, washermen, barbers, and etc on such wages as may be deemed unreasonable. The number of this description of servants which it may be necessary to entertain will of course be regulated by the future circumstances of the hospital and the number of patients.

5. The whole of the servants of the insane hospital, European as well as 'native' shall receive their pay from the department if the commissariat; and they shall be regularly mustered on the 1st day of each month by the visiting member of the medical board. The muster rolls in duplicate shall be prepared and attested in the usual manner one of these rolls shall be preserved by the commissariat and the other shall be forwarded to the military auditor general to enable that officer to audit the charges of the commissariat account of the servants of the establishment.

6. All the European servants of the insane hospitals shall be provided by the medical board in communication with the commissariat; and the power of discharging any of them for misconduct shall only be exercised by the medical board. All the 'native' servants required for the establishment shall be provided by the commissariat in communication with the surgeon of the hospital; who may discharge them when deemed necessary for misconduct.

7. Quarters will be provided for the surgeon and his assistant contiguous to the new insane hospital which it is intended to construct. Until the new hospital is completed those officers will procure accommodation as near as possible to the present hospital. The establishment of European servants above prescribed shall not be completed until quarters with which the present hospital is not provided, shall be constructed for them. The establishment of 'native' servants for the hospital shall be placed on the footing above described on the 1st of January next, when the general supply of that establishment shall be transferred to the commissariat; and at the same period all the rules above laid down shall be brought into operation, so far as may be found practicable under the present circumstances of that institution.

APPENDIX II: RULES FOR THE CONTROL AND MANAGEMENT OF THE HOUSE OF RECEPTION FOR EUROPEAN INSANE, MEDICAL CHARGE CONTROL AND SUPERINTENDENCE[2]

The general control superintendence of the house of reception for insane Europeans at this presidency is vested in the medical board and the magistrate of Calcutta.

The members of the medical board in succession and the first magistrate of Calcutta shall visit the house of reception together on the first day of every month and in those visits they will inspect minutely and make particular inquiries into the state of each patient. They will on the first day of each month, also submit to the govt. a return of the patients in the house of reception signed by them conjointly. With this return they will furnish a report containing their sentiments on the general state of the house of reception and on its management, in so far as regard the comfort and welfare of patients with reference to food, clothing, cleanliness, medical treatment, humane care and attention on the part of the surgeon of the house and those employed under his authority.

The following is the form of the monthly return which is to be submitted to the govt as above directed, viz. Names-Ranks-Admitted-Discharged-Died-Remarks.

Any of the magistrates of Calcutta and the members of the medical board shall visit the house as often as they may think it necessary. They will be held responsible that due care and attention are bestowed upon the patients every respect, and that no deficiency is permitted in regard to any object that may be conducive either to the welfare and comfort of their unhappy situation or to their ultimate recovery.

It will be the duty of the Medical Board to satisfy themselves that the house, which may be engaged by the superintendent for the reception of insane patients be so situated as to obviate in every practicable degree the chance of irritation to the patients from external objects.

Persons belonging to any of the corps of the army who are afflicted with the derangement shall be sent to the house of reception after having been examined and reported to be insane by a medical committee to be assembled for that purpose. Persons in the civil and marine departments will be admitted

[2] Medical Board Proceedings, Number 23, 13 April 1819, Enclosure to a letter sent to W. Ogilvy, President and Member of the Medical Board from C. Lushington, Secretary to Government in General Department, Council Chamber, dated 12 March 1819, NAI.

into the house after their insanity has been certified in respect to civil servants by two medical practitioners belonging to the service in Calcutta and in respect to the marine servants by the marine surgeon and his assistant. The insanity of persons unconnected with the public service shall in all practicable cases be certified by two medical practitioners before they are admitted into the house. The reports of medical committees in cases of insanity in the military department and the certificates in all the other several instances above mentioned, are to be transmitted to the surgeon of the house by whom they are to be carefully preserved. Transcripts and certificates are in every case to be made in a book of record which is to be kept at the house for that purpose and the authenticity of those copies is to be certified by the signature of the surgeon of the house.

All patients admitted into the house shall be visited and examined by a member of the medical board immediately on their admission or as soon afterwards as possible. That officer shall furnish the surgeon of the house with his opinion in writing respecting the person admitted with reference to the state of the malady, and the propriety of the future detention of the patient. The writing containing this opinion is to be carefully preserved by the surgeon of the house and a transcript of it to be made in the book of record above mentioned, immediately subjoined to the report or certificate relating to the sane patient. The authenticity of this copy is likewise to be certified by the signature of the surgeon of the house.

Patients shall be discharged from the house or sent on board ship for England only by the authority of the visiting member of the medical board. The sanction of govt in the latter case being of course previously obtained. In ordinary cases and in every instance when a patient is discharged or sent on board ship for England it will be necessary that the visiting member should previously furnish the surgeon on the house with his opinion in writing in respect to the propriety and safety of the discharge. This writing like those above mentioned will be carefully preserved and it shall be transcribed under a distinct head for patients discharged in the book of record which has been already described. This transcription shall likewise be authenticated in every instance by the signature of the surgeon of the house.

The members of the medical board and the first magistrate of Calcutta in all their monthly visits to the house shall carefully inspect this book of records and in their reports of govt shall state whether the above directions are duly and regularly complied with by the medical officer having the immediate charge of the house.

Besides these records it will be the duty of the surgeon of the house to keep a separate book in which the case of each patient if to be particularly described and the name period of admission, age, country, temperament, pursuits and habits of the patient and the history of the disease so far as it may be possible to ascertain those circumstances carefully detailed. The medical treatment and general management of each patient shall also from time to time be described in this book together with the success attending the measures adopted for the cure of the patient. In case of the bodily indisposition a daily report of the disease and its treatment shall be entered in this book, and in the events whether in death or in recovery stated as is usual in ordinary medical journals. The progressive result of the treatment for the cure of insanity, the periods of the disease of the patient, or in case of recovery those of the discharge shall also be carefully recorded.

The book shall be attentively inspected in the periodical visits of the members of the medical board and the first magistrate of Calcutta who in their reports to govt will state, whether this record is duly and regularly kept by the surgeon of the house.

The surgeon of the house shall furnish to the medical board a monthly return of his patients prepared according to the form above laid down for that which is to be submitted to the govt and this report shall be accompanied by a detail of all circumstances requiring the boards notice in any of the branches of the establishment.

The surgeon shall also furnish to be adjutant general of the army, for the information of his Excellency the commander in chief a quarterly return and report of all patients belonging to the military department who are in the house. The return will also be prepared according to the form above specified.

Whenever the members of the medical board in concurrence with the superintendent shall decide upon the propriety of sending a patient to Europe the surgeon shall address a letter upon the subject to the secretary to govt in the general department enclosing the opinion of that officer and stating the name, rank, age of the patient whereupon the govt shall see reason to concur in the propriety of its recommendation its sanction of the measure will be intimated by the secretary and the authority granted to the surgeon to secure a passage and provide (either personally or through the commissariat department) all requisite necessaries for such patient and to charge the amount of expense incurred in a contingent bill to be forwarded in the usual manner for the sanction of govt and audit.

It is not easy to fix the precise period of residence beyond which person labouring under insanity could no longer considered as fit objects of the house of reception but the establishment being in its nature one of purely temporary accommodation it may be generally considered that if after the expiration of six months from his admission a patient shall have shown no signs of approaching amendment the propriety of giving him a further chance of recovery by a removal to a colder climate may become a question of deliberation with the medical superintendents and that twelve months shall except under particular and unusual circumstances, be deemed the utmost length of time during which person shall be allowed to partake of the benefits of the institution.

Supply

The diet, clothing, bedding and all necessaries for the patients in the house (with the exception of medicines and surgical instruments) shall be supplied by the surgeon at the rate of 50 sicca rupees per mensem for each patient and he shall for this sum provide for each according to their previous rank.

As the adoption of precise rules in respect to the diet of the patients in the house of reception, would not appear to be practicable the quality and quantity of all articles of diet furnished must be regulated by the judgement and direction of the Surgeon of that establishment acting under the immediate control and superintendence of the medical board who will be held bound to see that the surgeon in every respect does justice to his patients and fulfils the obligations of his public duty.

All the supplies of wine and articles of that description shall be furnished an indent presented to the commissariat by the surgeon of the house and bearing the countersignature of the senior member of the medical board monthly statements shall be submitted to that board by the Surgeon of the house of the quantity of wine and other articles of that description expended in the house.

All the Europe and country medicines surgical instruments and apothecary utensils which are required for the house of reception shall be supplied from the honourable company's dispensary. Indent for such articles shall be prepared by the surgeon of the house according to the form prescribed by the general medical regulations for hospitals under this presidency. Their indents shall be submitted as often as necessary to the medical board by whom they will be examined and passed in the usual manner previously to their being complied with.

Servants

There shall be an European steward and apothecary in one person who shall reside at the house, and discharge his duties under the immediate direction and control of the surgeon of the house. This person shall receive a salary of 100 sicca rs. per month. There shall be also one head 'native' keeper at 12 sicca rupees per month. There ordinary 'native' keepers at 8 sicca rs. Each per month, one bhestee at 5 sicca rs. Per month, one metter at 5 sicca per month, and one tailor at 18 sicca rs. per month.

The whole of the servants of the house of reception European as well as 'native' shall receive their pay from the department of the commissariat and they shall be regularly mustered on the first day of each month by the visiting member of the medical board whose duty it shall be to ascertain that the whole of the establishment is regularly maintained. The muster roll in duplicate shall be prepared and attested in the usual manner. One of these rolls shall be preserved by the commissariat and the other shall be forwarded to the military auditor general to enable that officer to audit the charges of the commissariat on the account of the servants of the establishment

The surgeon of the house of reception shall provide all the servants European and 'native' and have power to discharge the sum on giving satisfactory reasons to the medical board.

APPENDIX III: THE RULES FOR PUBLIC AND PRIVATE PATIENTS ADMITTED AT BEARDSMORE'S PRIVATE ASYLUM[3]

Public Patients

1. Admission of insane in the army were sent to the asylum only after they were examined and reported to be insane by a medical committee specially made for the purpose. Persons in the civil and marine departments were admitted into the House after their insanity was certified. This certificate in case of the civil servants was produced by two medical practitioners attached to the service of the Honourable Company, and by the Marine Surgeon and his assistant in respect to marine servants.

2. The reports of medical committees and certificates of insanity in all the above instances were sent to the proprietor of the asylum. His responsibility was to preserve and transcript those documents in a book of record. The Surgeon verified it with a signature and also arranged for proper medical aid to the House.

3. The public patients were again divided into two classes, first, public patients of the better rank in life, and second, of common rank in life. The visiting member of the medical board determined this class division and charged the patients accordingly.

4. All bills for the maintenance of the public patients were countersigned by the visiting member of the medical board before the payment occurred at the general treasury.

Private Patients

1. On admission the insanity of all persons connected with the public service were certified by at least one medical practitioner and in all practicable cases two. Before they were admitted into the House such certificates were preserved as above and entered in the book of records.

2. All patients whether public or private admitted in the House were visited and examined by the visiting member of the medical board as soon as possible after admission. The officer furnished the proprietor of the House with his opinion in writing respecting the person admitted with reference to the state of his malady and propriety of his future detention. No person

[3] General Proceedings, General Department, Number 20, 13 July 1836, Letter sent to Beardsmore from James Jameson, Secretary Medical Board, dated 30 June 1821, WBSA.

was detained unless the opinion of the visiting member fully warranted the measure. The writing and the opinion of the visiting member were carefully preserved and recorded as above.

3. Public patients were discharged from the House only by the authority of the visiting member of the medical board who furnished the proprietor of the house with his opinion in writing on the propriety and safety of the discharge. These writings were carefully preserved and then entered into the book of records.

4. It was also desirable that no private patient be discharged without the previous advice and sanction of the visiting member.

5. No patient whether public or private were detained in the house after the visiting member and the surgeon of the house gave in their opinion that such person was fully restored to a sound state of mind.

6. It was extremely desirable that a separate book be kept by the attending surgeon in which the cases of all the patients shall be particularly described and the name, period of admission, age, country, temperament, pursuits, and habits of the patients and the history of the disease as far as ascertained be carefully detained. The medical treatment and general management of each patient, the success of the measures adopted for *his* care and the event of the disease whether in death or recovery. The period of decease or discharge were also noted.

7. The foregoing rule must be considered imperative in respect of the public patients and the book of cases be produced to the visiting member of the Board and the principal Magistrate of Calcutta at their periodical visits.

8. The proprietor of the House was supposed to furnish a weekly return of all the public patients under his charge to the Medical Board. These returns were countersigned by the attending Surgeon and from time to time were accompanied by a report of all circumstances requiring the Board's notice.

The following is the form of the weekly return.

FORM

Weekly Return of All Patients in the House of Reception for European Insane, Monday July 1821

Names	Ranks	Admitted	Died	Discharged	Remarks

9. Beside the weekly return he would also furnish a monthly return of all private patients in the House prepared according to the foregoing form.

10. On the first day of every month one of the members of the Medical Board in turn and the principal Magistrate of Calcutta visited the House together, minutely inspected and made particular enquiries into the state of each patient and it was expected that Mr. Beardmore would duly attend to all the remarks and suggestions, regarding the general management of the establishment and welfare of the patients which they thought proper to offer on such occasions.

11. Besides the above periodical visits, the several members of the Medical Board or their Secretary acting on their behalf would visit the asylum as often as they might think it necessary and would control and direct its general management. It would be the duty of the members of the Medical Board to superintendent the professional treatment of the patient to see that due care and attendance were paid to them in respect of accommodation, separation, diet, clothing, cleanliness, morals, humane care and that no deficiency was permitted (consistently with their relative conditions) in regard to any object that might be conducive either to the welfare and comfort or to their ultimate recovery.

12. In all cases of the proprietor would apply in the first instance to the visiting member and were the case was of sufficient importance to require it to the Medical Board through the channels of their Secretary.

The statistics of this asylum, which was a mere resting house for insane, few of whom live out of their insanity in it, were not of much value as compared with other institutions in which lunatics remained until they either recovered or died. Deaths, which occurred two in number, were of 'persons admitted in the extremity of illness', whom it was found impossible to restore. Bulk of the population consisted of soldiers, who were invalided for a condition of which the earlier stages were passed in regimental hospitals.[4]

[4] General Report Number 3 on the Lunatic Asylums, Vaccinations and Dispensaries in the Bengal Presidency for the Year 1870, compiled by Assistant Surgeon K. Macleod, A. M., M. D., Officiating Secretary to the Inspector General of Hospitals, Indian Medical Department (Calcutta: Bengal Secretariat Press, 1872).

GLOSSARY*

anna	the sixteenth part of a rupee
bheesty	water carrier
barkandaze	an armed retainer; an armed policeman, or other armed unmounted employee of a civil department
charas	a narcotic resin obtained from the flower heads of hemp
chiretta	a Himalayan herbaceous plant of the order *Gentianaceae* (*Swertia Chirata*)
dahi	curd
dhai	midwife
dhenkee	a pounding instrument used in villages to produce huskless paddy
dhobi	washerman
hakim	practitioner of Unani medicine
harkara	conveyer of news
jemadar	leader of a body of individuals
mali	gardener
mehtarnee	female sweeper

* The terms in the Glossary have been taken from Colonel Henry Yule and A. C. Burnell, *Hobson-Jobson: A Glossary of Colloquial Anglo Indian Words and Phrases, and of Kindred Terms, Etymological, Historical, Geographical and Discursive*, first published in 1886, new edition published in 1903 by W. Crooke (ed.), republished as the *Bengal Chamber Edition* on the occasion of the Tercentenary of Calcutta (Calcutta, Allahabad, Bombay, Delhi: Rupa and Company, 1990).

mehtar	sweeper
morah	stool; a footstool
naib	deputy
peon	originally used in the sense of 'a foot soldier', then an 'orderly' or messenger
pice	*paisā*, a small copper coin, which under the Anglo-Indian system of currency is one-fourth of an anna, or the sixty-fourth part of a rupee
pukka	cemented
soorky	pounded brick used to mix with lime to form a hydraulic mortar
Sudder Adalat	district court
tat	kind of mat
24 Parganas	official name of the district immediately adjoining and enclosing, though not administratively including, Calcutta
vaid	practitioners of Ayurvedic medicine

SELECT BIBLIOGRAPHY

ARCHIVAL SOURCES

National Archives of India, New Delhi

Annual Reports of the Asylums of Bengal, 1856–85
Government of Bengal, Medical Board Proceedings, 1798–1855
Government of Bengal, Public Works Department Proceedings, 1850–5
Government of India, Home (Medical) Proceedings, 1830–40
Government of India, Home (Public) Proceedings, 1825–35
Government of India, Municipal (Medical) Proceedings, 1890–1900
Native Newspaper Reports, Bengal, 1887–95

Asia, Pacific and Africa Collection, British Library, London

Government of Bengal, Criminal (Judicial) Proceedings, 1805–20
Government of Bengal, Home (Medical) Proceedings, 1855–70
Government of Bengal, Municipal (Medical) Proceedings, 1890–1900

West Bengal State Archives, Kolkata

Government of Bengal, Criminal (Judicial) Proceedings, 1805–20
Government of Bengal, General (General) Proceedings, 1830–45
Government of Bengal, General (Medical) Proceedings, 1860–70
Government of Bengal, Judicial (Criminal) Proceedings, 1805–20

National Library, Kolkata

Rare Books Collections

Wellcome Institute for the History of Medicine, London

Asylum Journals
Monthly Journal of Medical Science

SECONDARY SOURCES

Published before 1900

Bucknill, John Charles. 'Report on East Indian Asylums.' *The Asylum Journal of Mental Sciences*, 5 (1858–9): 218–222.

———, ed. *Asylum Journal of Mental Sciences*. London: Association of Medical Officers of Asylums and Hospitals for the Insane, 1855.

Bucknill, John Charles, and Daniel Hack Tuke, eds. *A Manual of Psychological Medicine: Containing the History, Nosology, Description, Statistics, Diagnosis, Pathology and Treatment of Insanity, with an Appendix of Cases*. London: John Churchill, 1862.

Conolly, John. *The Construction and Government of Lunatic Asylums and Hospitals for the Insane*. London: John Churchill, 1847.

Cox, Joseph Mason. *Practical Observations on Insanity; in which Some Suggestions are Offered Towards an Improved Mode of Treating Diseases of the Mind and Some Rules Proposed which it is Hoped May Lead to a More Humane and Successful Method of Cure: to Which are Subjoined Remarks on Medical Jurisprudence as it Relates to Diseased Intellect*. London: R. Baldwin and T. Underwood, 1813.

Curie, James. *Medical Reports on the Effects of Water Cold and Warm, as a Remedy in Fever and Febrile Diseases, whether Applied to the Surface of the Body, or used Internally*. Liverpool: J. M. Creery, 1804.

Greene, W. A. 'Contributions towards the Pathology of Insanity in India'. *The Annals of Medical Science* 4 (1857): 374–435.

Hill, Robert Gardiner. *A Concise History of the Entire Abolition of Mechanical Restraint in the Treatment of the Insane; and of the Introduction, Success, and Final Triumph of the Non Restraint System, together with a Reprint of a Lecture Delivered on the Subject in the Year 1838 and Appendices, containing an Account of the Controversies and Claims Connected therewith*. London: Longman, Brown, Green, and Longmans, 1857.

Hill, Robert Gardiner. 'On the Non Restraint System.' In *Asylum Journal of Mental Sciences*, edited by John Charles Bucknill, Number 10, January 1855, 153–5. London: Association of Medical Officers of Asylums and Hospitals for the Insane, 1855.

Leeuwen, H. Van. 'On the Medico and Moral Treatment of Insanity.' In *Asylum Journal of Mental Sciences*, edited by John Charles Bucknill, Volume 2, Number 6, July 1, 1854, 91–3. London: Association of Medical Officers of Asylums and Hospitals for the Insane, 1855.

Martin, James Ronald. *Influence of Tropical Climates on European Constitutions.* Calcutta, Military Orphan Press, 1841.

———. *Notes on Medical Topography of Calcutta.* Calcutta: Military Orphan Press, 1837.

Medico Psychological Association. *Handbook for the Instruction of Attendants on the Insane.* Boston: Cupples, Upham, and Company, 1886.

Mercier, Charles. *The Attendants Companion: A Manual of the Duties of Attendants in Lunatic Asylums.* London: J. & A. Churchill, 1898.

Moore, W. J. *A Manual of the Diseases in India.* London: John Churchill, 1861.

Reid, James. 'On the Symptoms, Causes and Treatment of Puerperal Insanity.' In *Asylum Journal of Mental Sciences*, edited by John Charles Bucknill, Volume 2, 1855–6.

Tuke, Daniel Hack, ed. *A Dictionary of Psychological Medicine: Giving the Definition, Etymology and Synonyms of the Terms Used in Medical Psychology with the Symptoms, Treatment, and Pathology of Insanity and the Law of Lunacy in Great Britain and Ireland*, volume 2. London: J. & A. Churchill, 1892.

———. *Moral Management of the Insane and the Various Contrivances which have been Adopted Instead of Mechanical Restraint.* London: John Churchill, 1854.

———. 'On the Various Forms of Mental Disorder.' In *Asylum Journal of Mental Sciences*, edited by John Charles Bucknill, Volume 3, 1856–7.

Tuke, Samuel. *Description of the Retreat, an Institution Near York for Insane Persons of the Society of Friends Containing an Account of its Origin and Progress, the Modes of Treatment, and a Statement of Cases.* London: Society of Friends, 1813.

Wise, Alexander Thomas. 'Principle Remarks on Insanity as it Occurs Among the Inhabitants of Bengal.' *Monthly Journal of Medical Science* 15 (July–December 1852).

Published after 1900

Appignanesi, Lisa. *Mad, Bad and Sad: A History of Women and the Mind Doctors from 1800 to the Present.* London: Virago, 2008.

Arnold, David. *The New Cambridge History of India, Science, Technology and Medicine in Colonial India*. Cambridge: Cambridge University Press, 2000.

Bala, Poonam. *Imperialism and Medicine in Bengal: A Socio-Historical Perspective*. New Delhi, Newbury Park, London: Sage, 1991.

Bynum, William F. 'Rationales for Therapy in British Psychiatry, 1780–1835'. *Medical History* 18, no. 4 (1964): 317–34.

Bynum, William F., Roy Porter, and Michael Shepherd, eds. *The Anatomy of Madness*, Volume 2. London: Tavistock, 1985.

Chesler, Phyllis. *Women and Madness*. New York: Palgrave Macmillan, 2005.

Digby, Anne. *Madness, Mortality and Medicine: A Study of the York Retreat, 1796–1914*. Cambridge: Cambridge University Press, 1985.

Edginton, Barry. 'A Space for Moral Management: The York Retreat's Influence on Asylum Design,' in *Madness, Architecture and the Built Environment, Psychiatric Spaces in Historical Context*, edited by Leslie Topp, James E. Moran, and Jonathan Andrews. New York: Routledge, 2007.

Ernst, Waltraud. 'Asylum Provision and the East Indian Company in the Nineteenth Century.' *Medical History* 42 (1998): 476–502.

———. 'European Madness and Gender in Nineteenth-Century British India.' *Social History of Medicine* 9, no. 3 (1996): 357–82.

———. 'Feminising Madness - Feminising the Orient: Madness, Gender and Colonialism in British India, 1860–1940.' In *Exploring Gender Equations: Colonial and Post Colonial India*, edited by Biswamoy Pati and Shakti Kak. New Delhi: Nehru Memorial Museum and Library, 2005.

———. 'Idioms of Madness and Colonial Boundaries the Case of the European and "Native" Mentally Ill in Early Nineteenth Century British India.' *Comparative Studies in Society and History* 39, no. 1 (January 1997): 153–81.

———. 'Institutions, People and Power: Lunatic Asylums in Bengal, 1800–1900.' In *The Social History of Health and Medicine in Colonial India*, edited by Biswamoy Pati and Mark Harrison, 129–50. Oxford: Routledge, 2009.

———. 'Madness and Colonial Spaces—British India, c. 1800–1947.' In *Madness, Architecture and Built Environment, Psychiatric Spaces in Historical Context*, edited by Leslie Topp, James E. Moran, and Jonathan Andrews. New York: Routledge, 2007.

———. *Mad Tales from the Raj: The European Insane in British India, 1800-1858*. London: Routledge, 1991.

Foucault, Michel. *Madness and Civilization: A History of Insanity in the Age of Reason*, translated by Richard Howard. New York: Vintage Books, 1965.

Goffman, Erving. *Asylums: Essays on the Social Situation of Mental Patients and Other Inmates*. New York: Anchor Books, 1961.

Harrison, Mark. *Climates and Constitutions: Health, Race, Environment and British Imperialism in India, 1600–1850*. New York: Oxford University Press, 1999.

———. 'Morbid Anatomy in British India, 1770–1850.' In *The Social History of Health and Medicine in Colonial India*, edited by Biswamoy Pati and Mark Harrison, 173–94. Oxford: Routledge, 2009.

Hide, Louise. *Gender and Class in English Asylums, 1890–1914*. Basingstoke: Palgrave Macmillan, 2014.

Ingram, Allan, ed. *Patterns of Madness in the Eighteenth Century: A Reader*. Liverpool: Liverpool University Press, 1998.

Keller, Richard. 'Madness and Colonization: Psychiatry in the British and French Empires, 1800–1962.' *Journal of Social History* 35, no. 2 (Winter 2001): 295–326.

Kumar, Deepak and Raj Sekhar Basu, eds. *Medical Encounters in British India*. New Delhi: Oxford University Press, 2013.

Marland, Hilary. *Dangerous Motherhood: Insanity and Childbirth in Victorian Britain*. Basingstoke: Palgrave Macmillan, 2004.

Mills, James. *Madness, Cannabis and Colonialism: The 'Native-Only' Lunatic Asylums of British India, 1857–1900*. Basingstoke: Macmillan, 2000.

———. '"More Important to Civilise than Subdue?" Lunatic Asylums, Psychiatric Practice and Fantasies of "the Civilising Mission" in British India 1858–1900.' In *Colonialism as Civilising Mission: Cultural Ideology in British India*, edited by Harald Fischer-Tiné and Michael Mann, 179–90. London: Anthem South Asian Studies, 2004.

———. 'The History of Modern Psychiatry in India 1858–1947.' *History of Psychiatry*, xii (2001): 431–58.

Noll, Richard. *The Encyclopaedia of Schizophrenia and Other Psychotic Disorders*. New York: Facts on File, 1992 (third edition, accessed on Google Books in November 2010).

Pati, Biswamoy and Mark Harrison, eds. *The Social History of Health and Medicine in Colonial India*. London and New York: Routledge, 2009.

Porter, Roy. *Madmen: A Social History of Madhouses, Mad Doctors and Lunatics*. Stroud, Gloucestershire: Tempus, 2004.

———. *Madness: A Brief History*. Oxford: Oxford University Press, 2002.

———, ed. *Medicine in the Enlightenment*. Amsterdam and Atlanta, GA: Rodopi, 1995.

Ripa, Yannick. *Women and Madness: The Incarceration of Women in Nineteenth Century France*, translated by Catherine du Peloux Menage. Cambridge: Polity Press, 1990.

Scull, Andrew. *The Most Solitary of Afflictions: Madness and Society in Britain 1700–1900*. New Haven, London: Yale University Press, 1993.

Sen, Indrani. 'The Memsahib's "Madness": The European Woman's Mental Health in Late Nineteenth Century India.' *Social Scientist* 33, no. 5–6 (May–June 2005): 26–48.

Showalter, Elaine. *The Female Malady: Women, Madness, and English Culture, 1830–1980*. London: Virago Press, 1987.

Smith, Leonard. 'The Architecture of Confinement: Urban Asylums in England, 1750–1820.' In *Madness, Architecture and the Built Environment: Psychiatric Spaces in Historical Context*, edited by Leslie Topp, James E. Moran, and Jonathan Andrews. New York: Routledge, 2007.

Szasz, Thomas S. *The Manufacture of Madness: A Comparative Study of the Inquisition and the Mental Health Movement*. London: Routledge and Kegan Paul, 1971.

———. *The Myth of Mental Illness: Foundation of a Theory of Personal Conduct*. New York: Perennial Library Edition, 1974.

Topp, Leslie, James E. Moran, and Jonathan Andrews, eds. *Madness, Architecture and the Built Environment: Psychiatric Spaces in Historical Context*. New York: Routledge, 2007.

INDEX

Association of Medical Officers of
Asylums and Hospitals for Insane
in England, 95
asthenia, 148, 155
mortality to, 156–60
Asylum Journal, 95
asylum physicians, comparison
between Britain and India, 5
asylums of Bengal, colonial era, 5.
See also Berhampore Lunatic
Asylum; Dacca Lunatic Asylum;
Moorshedabad Lunatic Asylum;
Moydapore Lunatic Asylum; Patna
Lunatic Asylum; Russapaglah
(Dullunda) Lunatic Asylum
assessment of causes of mental
illness, 22–4
Assistant Surgeon of an asylum, 17
condition for admittance, 22
diversity in practices of superintendents, 26–7
Ernst's work on, 5
gender issues, 6–7
increase/decrease in asylum
population, reasons for, 29–34

location of, 34
magistrate, empowerment in
admissions and discharges,
17–19
medical history sheets, 27
medical officers' involvement with
issues of insanity, 21
notions of masculinity and
femininity, 6–7
overcrowding in, 31–2
provincial medical boards of
1780s, 16
race and class divisions, issues of,
5–6
rules for payment, 32–3
rules for the management of,
238
rules of admission to, 32
scope for post-treatment observation of patients, 21
social composition and condition
of patients, 20
space allotted to the inmates, 29
staff attendance, 17
superintendents of, 16–17, 19

servants of, 267–8
supply to, 267

infirm gang, 28
insane hospitals, 2
insanity, definition of, 2–3, 14–29, 138
    differences of categorization of
        insanity, 25
    due to consumption of intoxicat-
        ing substances, 25, 155, 161–2
    due to overcrowding, 163–4
    as exaltation of emotion, 26
    infirm gang, 28
    'intellectual and emotional'
        causes, 24, 140
    nomenclatures for classifying
        mental illness, 24–5
Inspector General of Hospitals, 19,
    21, 26, 28, 31, 59, 239, 245–6
institutionalized lunatics, 134–5

*Journal of Psychological Medicine and
    Mental Pathology*, 95

lunatic asylums, 2–3
    works by historians, 9–10

Medical Board, 15–17, 19, 36–7,
    40–4, 46, 62, 75, 85, 99, 123,
    171, 173–4, 177
medical therapies, 93–105, 196
    before and after 1858, 95
    apothecaries and physicians'
        duties, 93–4
    application of 'setons' on the
        neck, 99
    bathing, 96–7
    bloodlettings and other cathartics,
        94, 96, 102
    blue pills along with castor oil, 99
    circulations on a swing, 97

counter irritants (croton oil, tarter
    emetic ointment, and liniment
    iodine), 104
decoction of bark with sulphuric
    acid, sulphate of quinine, and
    sulphate of iron, 100
effect of the moon and, 96
eighteenth-century, 94
frog soup, 104
Hindu medicine, 104
hygienic treatment, 99
iodine, 100
mixture of camphor, 96
opium therapy, 98
port wine with quinine, 104
purgatives and doses of antimony,
    96, 100
regulation of bowels, 102
sedatives and tonics, 100
sulphate of cinchonidine, iron,
    and sulphuric acid, 105
Unani medicine, 104–5
using leeches, 98, 100–1
using narcotics and tincture, 103
medico-moral treatment, 76–8
*mehtarnee*s, 194
mental illnesses in India
    GOI awareness campaign, 1–2
    non-government organizations,
        role in treatment, 16
Moorshedabad Lunatic Asylum, 45,
    60–7, 215
    cases of mania among female
        inmates, 170
    convalescent wards, 64
    idea of separate cells, 64–5
    method of treatment, 65
    modifications to construction,
        66–7
    mortality rates, 67
    number of cells, 64, 66

ABOUT THE AUTHOR

Debjani Das is Assistant Professor, Department of History, Vidyasagar University, West Bengal, India. She works on the social history of medicine in colonial India.